D1808276

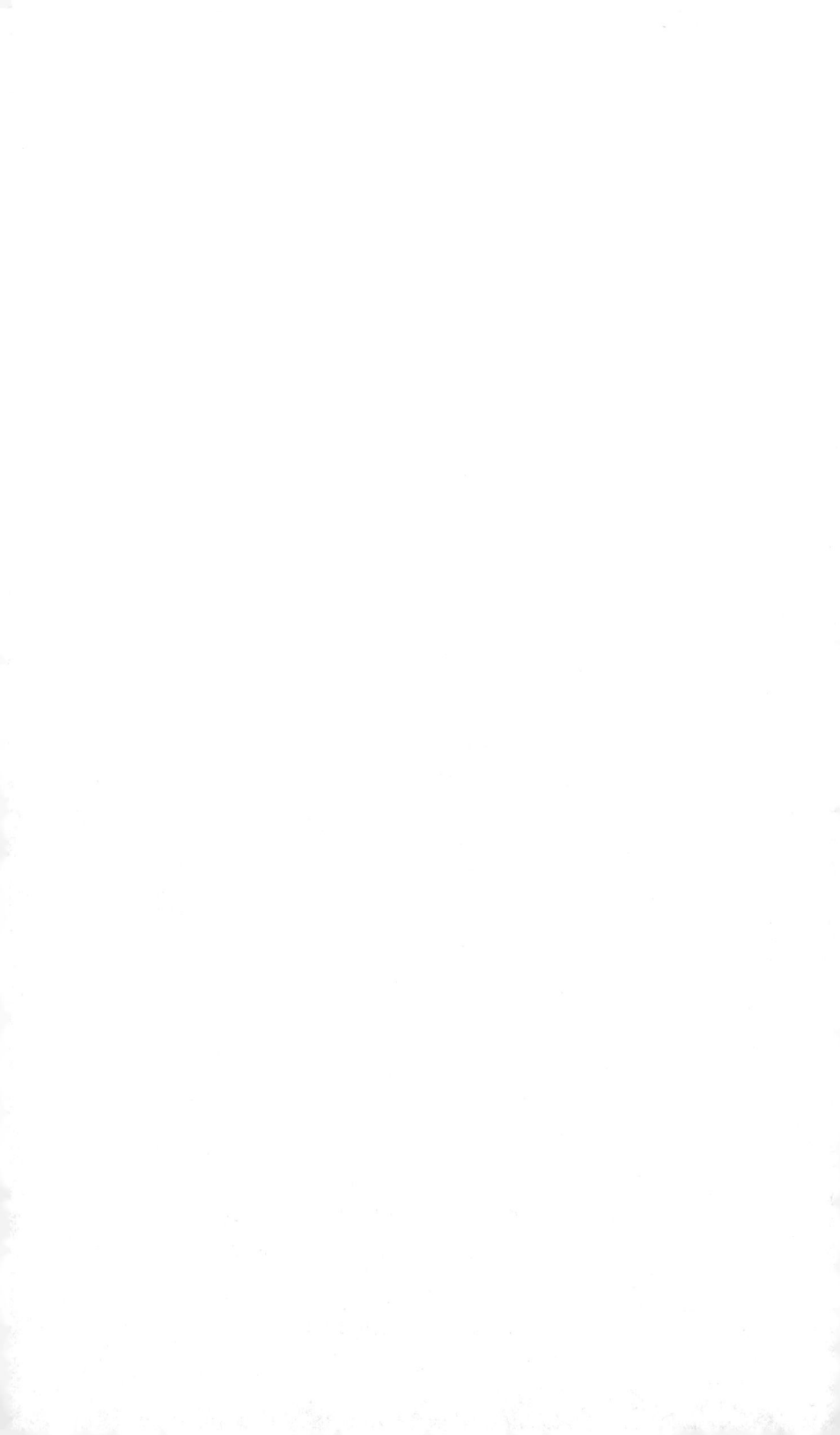

Conquering Kids' Cancer

Triumphs and Tragedies of a Children's Cancer Doctor

Kenneth Lazarus, M.D.

Copyright January© 1999 by Emerald Ink Publishing
All rights reserved.

Published by:

Emerald Ink Publishing
9700 Almeda-Genoa Rd.
Suite 502
Houston, Texas 77087

(800) 324-5663

E-mail emerald@emeraldink.com
http://www.emeraldink.com

Printed and bound in the United States of America

Library of Congress Cataloging-in-Publication Data

Lazarus, Kenneth 1951-
  Conquering Kids' Cancer: triumphs and tragedies of a
children's cancer doctor / Kenneth H. Lazarus
  p. cm.
  Includes bibliographical references (p. 2) and index.
  ISBN 1-885373-22-8 (pbk.)
  1. Tumors in children. I. Title.
  RC281.C4 L39 1999
  618.92'994--dc21

                    98-40258
                      CIP

Dedication

This book is dedicated to my wife, Marian, who is the best friend and nurse I could ever have and to my wonderful, bright, and supportive children, Melissa and Stephanie. My love and thanks go out to my mother-in-law Anna, sister-in-law, Bella, nephew, Craig and niece, Michelle.

I also send my love and devotion to all of the children and their parents, siblings, grandparents, aunts, uncles, cousins and friends whom I have been so privileged to get to know over the years.

Introduction

To cure sometime,
To relieve often,
To comfort always.

15th century folk saying

The past decade has witnessed miraculous breakthroughs in our understanding and treatment of childhood cancers. Through the dedicated efforts of basic scientists and clinical researchers, we can now confidently talk about "cure" for many children diagnosed with malignant diseases. Furthermore, the treatment process itself has become much more humane—both for the children undergoing treatment and for their families. Problems with painful procedures, nausea and vomiting are largely a thing of the past. The future holds even more breakthroughs. By unlocking the genetic basis of specific cancers, we will be able to switch off cancer-promoting genes and switch on self-destruct genes in the cancer cells themselves. These very specific treatments will soon allow us to do away with our current "primitive" cancer-treating tools, including chemotherapy and radiation therapy. Future genetic therapies promise to be much more tolerable and much more effective.

Ironically, these advances in the science of medicine have coincided with an all-pervasive deterioration in the art of medicine. Many factors are responsible for this "dehumanizing" of health care. These factors all have in common the distancing of physicians from their patients. For example, the majority of physicians are now employed by large health care conglomerates which control the "how, when and where" of patient care. There is little room in this schema for the physician to listen to the patient on a personal level. Both doctor and patient (or "provider" and "client" to use the corporate jargon) often feel like cogs on a wheel in a machine on an assembly line.

This model of practice must change. In this book, by example after poignant example, Dr. Lazarus tells us not how to enact the change, but rather what the change should look like. He paints a picture of the true healer—one who combines the best of medical science with deep respect and loving kindness.

Nathan L. Kobrinsky, M.D.

Roger Maris Cancer Center
Fargo, North Dakota

Contents

Notes from the Publisher

Introduction *by Nathan L. Kobrinsky, M.D.*

More Than A Disease

The happy noises and the general chaos in the small room belied the reason the children and their families were sitting there. Two of the children had very little hair, but no one seemed to notice. Bright cartoon pictures of bears engaged in various activities decorated the walls. The doors of a toy closet in one corner of the room had been flung open—toys and games covered the floor. At a small table next to the closet, three children of different ages were trying to build a tower out of blocks and a fourth was having a play battle with plastic soldiers. On the other side of the toy closet, a mother and father sat beside their teenaged son. He had a baseball cap on his head with the brim set backwards. He wore a slightly disapproving smirk. His mother was smiling at the antics of the children at the game table. On the opposite side of the room, a young woman with short, curly blonde hair was trying to reason with her 2-year old in what was clearly a losing battle. Another mother was holding her infant in her arms in the chair next to the frustrated mother. A second teenager in a private school uniform sat in the adjacent chair. Her arms were folded and her legs were crossed at the ankles, but there was a smile on her face. Two young parents sat on the floor while their toddlers played happily in front of them.

As I gazed over the group, I noticed two families standing outside in the hall, either to escape the hubbub or because they realized that there was just no way for more people to squeeze into the small room. I realized that I knew the people in that reception area better than I knew some members of my own family. I knew which parents were having marital or financial problems, which were planning to move and which had a fairly stable and enjoyable life. I knew which children were outstanding students and which were just scraping by. In many instances, I knew the names of their dogs or cats and how many years those pets had been a part of the family.

I had become more than the doctor. These people were my friends.

Few people looking in on the happy faces would have realized that about half of the children in that room that day were being treated for some sort of cancer. Some could be identified by their wispy or absent hair, but most were indistinguishable from any other child. Many of the children called out my name when they saw me, and a few ran up to hug me. Some just wanted to say hello and some wanted to tell me about the game they were playing or about how school was going. Some were shy or even a little scared but a wave or a touch or a kiss would usually bring a smile.

Each child was called by name to come back to the treatment room. For some, I would sing and dance while I examined them. With the younger ones I would bark or meow when I looked in their ears and then act surprised that they had animals in their ears. The older children would tell me that I was being silly, because they knew that I was making the funny noises. Some of the younger children would ask what was in their ears that day or even tell me which specific animals were in which ear.

Some children would sit quietly and shyly. There were a few that never spoke to me and after a while their silence would become our joke. Some would run around playing and have to be captured for their examination. Others would tease me about my balding hair and I would feign shock or dismay. Marian (my wife and nurse) and I almost always worked right through lunch, but we never (or hardly ever) noticed. Each child was special and important. We could never spend enough time with each one.

At one point, each of these children and their families had been unknown to me. The children had developed symptoms that had brought them to the attention of their parents or family physician. I had subsequently been called in once it had been determined that the source of their symptoms was a cancer of some sort. What had begun as a frightening, almost overwhelming situation had become for the children, their families and myself almost a daily routine and we had developed far more than a doctor-patient relationship.

Why did I write this book? I think it is because I have observed the medical system from the inside. I have been a consumer myself so I have seen the good and the bad of medicine from both sides. I have a strong belief in the role of emotional support in the healing process, but I do not espouse "alternative" treatments. The scientific method is the best way to prove that medical therapies are effective and safe. However, in our zeal to treat, we must never forget that we are treating more than a disease.

I entered medical school in 1973 fresh from college. My undergraduate degree was in psychology. I thought I would go to medical school to become a psychiatrist. Several events that occurred white I was in medical school not only convinced me that psychiatry was not right for me but also profoundly influenced my thinking. Even today, I recall those occasions for their impact on my philosophy of life and of medicine.

At the end of my first year of medical school, I was totally unprepared for anything medical. The courses I had taken that first year had taught me only general structure and function of the human body. Such courses included anatomy, histology, pharmacology, physiology and biochemistry. In order to finance my way through medical school, I had enrolled in an Air Force scholarship program. The Air Force paid for my medical school tuition and books. In return, I agreed to serve in the military one year for every year that had been paid.

Part of the agreement was that I would spend 45 days each summer at an Air Force base as an *extern*. An *extern* is a medical student who is under the guidance of an experienced physician something like a student driver. By a series of coincidences, I ended up spending my time the first summer in pediatrics with a pediatric *nephrologist* (a kidney specialist) as my mentor. This doctor was and still is my vision of the consummate pediatrician. He was warm, caring and loving with the children and their families. He was exceedingly bright and challenged me to use my meager knowledge to think through clinical problems. I left the Air Force base that summer when my 45-day tour of duty was completed with a great appreciation of pediatrics. I was not sure if my feelings toward the field were due to my respect for my teacher or because I truly liked children. I also returned to my second year of medical school with an appreciation for how important each bit of information that I had learned so painstakingly in my first year would be in my future endeavors.

The next summer I returned to the same Air Force base for my second externship. This time pediatrics was the chosen field for my 45-day obligation. The pediatric nephrologist whom I so admired was getting ready to leave the Air Force since he had nearly completed his commitment. As a result, he was less available than he had been the year before. The second summer externship turned out to be as important to me as the one before, if not more so.

While serving my time, I met two children on the pediatric ward who confirmed my love of pediatrics and who probably had a little to do with my eventual choice of subspecialties. Andy was a cute 18-month old boy who had been sick for about one week. Acute Lymphocytic Leukemia (ALL) was diagnosed after his mother brought him to the pediatric clinic to find out why he was not getting better. I had little to do with him from a medical standpoint, but I spent several mornings that summer talking with his mother about her feelings. I gained a strong idea of the anger, loss of control, fear and disbelief that such a diagnosis brings to a family. I do not know what happened to Andy. I hope that he has turned out to be one of the thousands of children now cured of ALL, but I am grateful to him and his mother for their willingness to share so deeply with me so many years ago.

I was most profoundly affected by Bobby, an 8-year old with ALL, who had already suffered two recurrences of the leukemia in the bone marrow. Bobby was chubby from the medications that were used in the treatment of leukemia. He was almost always happy. When I was assigned Bobby as the patient I was to follow, I remember walking past his room thinking that he did not want to talk to me. When I reached the end of the hall, I realized that Bobby had not said a single word to me. My problem was that *I* was afraid to get to know *him*.

With that insight, I marched into his room and introduced myself. Bobby turned out to be a special young man. I would spend one to two hours every day in his room. We rarely talked about the leukemia. He liked to play cards or build things with blocks that snapped together. He would tell me stories about hunting for frogs or fishing at a lake near his rural home using worms he had dug up in the family garden. Bobby had great ideas about what he wanted to do in the future without knowing, or maybe because he did know, that his future was extremely limited. His disease continued to progress during the 45 days of my externship. He died on the day I was scheduled to leave and return to my third year of medical school. I went to the hospital room where he and I had spent so many happy hours together looking out at the sunshine and talking about a future that did not even exist. The windows were darkened by closed drapes and the mood was somber and sad. I hugged Bobby's grieving parents and silently said good-bye to my young friend. As I drove home later that day, I inwardly thanked Bobby because he had taught me so much about myself and about how to live. Bobby taught me about the dignity of life—and of death.

I have often thought how valuable and meaningful his short life had been. Bobby taught me the very valuable lesson about *the importance of maintaining a person's dignity* even when they are ill. There comes a time in medical school when one must give up the relative safety of the lecture hall and the laboratory and learn how to interview and examine real live people. This experience can be intimidating to students who up until that time have relied on a good memory or a book to carry them through. One event stands out vividly.

One day while I was standing on one of the wards of the medical school's teaching hospital waiting with my fellow students for our instructor, a senior medical student burst through the door and shouted, "Where is that *embolus* in bed three?"

I turned toward the third bed fully expecting to see a giant blood clot sitting in the middle of the bed. In that one statement, that fourth year student had reduced that patient's life to the disease which had brought him to the hospital. I vowed that I would try to never trivialize a person's life nor devalue their emotions like that medical student had.

This lesson was further driven home to me when I was hospitalized for a minor surgical procedure a few months later. The experience was dehumanizing and embarrassing. I felt like a slab of meat pushed and pulled from one venue to another with no control over what was happening to me. My self-esteem was shaken by the experience. How can one get better in such an environment? It is a shame that more medical personnel do not get a chance to experience the other side of medical care. Perhaps, then, there would be more appreciation of the emotional difficulties produced by illness.

While these experiences convinced me that children and I were made for each other and that there was a dignified, personal way to treat them, I still did not know in which branch of pediatrics I wanted to spend the rest of my working life. Being a lover of knowledge, I liked virtually every aspect of the field. One of my favorite residents while I was an intern told me that she was planning to study childhood cancer. It seemed like such a good idea that I began to look into it.

My future in pediatric oncology was settled one late December afternoon during the second year of my post-graduate training. As a resident we were entitled to only two weeks of vacation each year. Since we worked 80 to 100 hours each week, we treasured every extra moment we could arrange off.

During the Christmas season each year the hospital would be relatively empty so that as many children as possible could be home with their families. Only the sickest children remained behind. Since the workload was usually lighter, one-half of the residents would work during the week of Christmas while the other half took off. When the vacationing group returned from their short but welcome break, the residents who had worked the Christmas week would then take their week off. I always worked the Christmas week because I was Jewish and because it was usually quieter during the Christmas week than the week which followed. Christmas Eve day that year was unusually quiet.

I was assigned to cover the fourth floor, which included the oncology and endocrinology wards. Around two in the afternoon, I asked the intern who was responsible for the oncology ward to gather up those children with cancer who had remained in the hospital and bring them to the playroom. By half past two the room was filled with children, siblings, parents, nurses, and two slightly nervous, neophyte pediatricians. Only one child was too ill to leave his room. For two hours that afternoon, we sang all of the Christmas carols we could think of. We laughed whenever we could not remember the words to a song, which was not terribly infrequent. After all, does anyone really know all the words to, "Good King Wenceslaus"? It was a marvelous and magical afternoon. It brought some cheer to a dreary place to spend a special holiday and made my career choice much easier.

All of these experiences and many more have contributed to teaching me the values and integrity I cherish as a physician and as a human being. My years in a fellowship learning the ins and outs of the field of pediatric oncology were followed by the four years I owed to the Air Force for my scholarship to medical school. During my four years on active duty, I was able to practice my chosen field of pediatric hematology/oncology. The four years passed too quickly. During that time I learned more about my field and acquired valuable experience. Although I worked hard, I know that I got the better of the deal when I joined the Air Force and received a scholarship to medical school. I would have stayed in the Air Force if there had been more support for pediatrics, but the Air Force medical system was established to provide support to military personnel and not to their dependents. I fully understood why pediatrics did not rate higher.

During the fourth and final year of my Air Force service, a profoundly important event made many changes in my life and allowed me to understand my chosen field and myself much better. My wife's sister developed leukemia. It was the evening before Thanksgiving. Marian and I had planned to have four couples over for a feast the next day. Marian was 8 months pregnant and it had not been an easy pregnancy. I had gone to the store to get some last minute supplies. Marian stayed home with our 2-year old daughter and got her ready for bed. I returned from shopping about an hour later. When I walked through the door, I found Marian distraught and in tears. I had only seen Marian cry once before, so I knew something horrible must have happened.

"What's going on?" I asked, frantic to find out that everything was okay with my daughter, my wife, and the unborn baby. "Take a deep breath and tell me what happened."

After a few suffocated sobs, she replied, "My sister called. She said she had developed this strange rash on her ankles when she came home from a business trip to Hawaii. She thought it might be a sun reaction, but when it did not go away, she went to her doctor. Her blood count is real abnormal. Her doctor told her it might be an infection, but I know that she has leukemia."

The news had indeed been horrible. It was too late to cancel the Thanksgiving party. The next day we entertained our friends and the day somehow passed. Thanksgiving that year was not much of a celebration since we now had little to celebrate. By the day after Thanksgiving my sister-in-law knew what we had realized two days earlier. She really did have leukemia. She called us in tears and told us that her doctor had said that she had the worst kind of leukemia and that she would be dead in less than one week. I am not sure that those were that doctor's exact words or even his sentiments, but that was the message Bella had heard.

We told her we would arrange for her to come to our house, and we would find someone to take care of her leukemia who would have a more positive view. The very next day my sister-in-law, my teenage nephew and niece, and my mother-in-law arrived at the airport. In just three days my sister-in-law had changed from a vibrant woman with an unusual rash to someone who was terribly weak and could barely walk. She needed a wheelchair to help her get off the plane. I had contacted a doctor friend of mine who took care of adults with cancer. He had agreed to help in Bella's care. We drove straight from the airport to the hospital. It was a strange feeling to be a brother-in-law and not the doctor. Once we reached the hospital, the nurses and technicians snapped quickly into action. Blood was drawn and IV's were started. Within 24 hours of arrival, chemotherapy was flowing into her veins. The first hospitalization lasted three weeks.

I recall checking Bella out of the hospital. I went to the discharge cashier's office with the form the nurses had given me. The cashier, in a flat, unemotional voice, said, "That will be $19,513.17, please."

I reached for my wallet before I realized the absurdity of her request. I answered in a very cheery voice, "I am so sorry. I left my money at home in my other pants."

The cashier did not smile at my comment. Instead she stamped something on the form and handed it back with a disapproving look on her face. Two weeks after Bella developed leukemia, my younger daughter, Stephanie, was born. The delivery was uneventful but the problems that had followed Marian during the pregnancy continued after the delivery. Marian needed surgery before she could come home. The two sisters were managed in different hospitals in different parts of the city. I remember going from one hospital to the other in a semi-fugue state. I tried to make some sense of my life, but everything seemed topsy-turvy. Having a newborn baby was supposed to be a joyous time, but I had not had a chance to enjoy my new daughter. Once my wife got better, all her free time was spent in the hospital with her sister. The baby slept on a spare bed in the hospital room while Marian helped her sister through the fevers and nausea and body aches of the leukemia and its treatment.

My house, the first one I had ever owned, was now filled. My mother-in-law could barely function because she was so filled with grief and fear. My niece was having difficulty dealing with her mother's illness. She tried to continue work and her college education, but she had difficulty dealing with her anger. She would be home for only brief moments because of her busy schedule, but we still received much of her pent-up rage. Fortunately, she loved helping with the newborn baby and her 2-year old cousin, and the babies helped take her focus off her miserable situation.

My nephew had to be re-enrolled in a new and strange high school. He resented being uprooted from his home and his friends. He further resented the fact that his uncle and aunt had taken on the role of father and mother. He was a good young man with strong values, but he kept his anger and confusion hidden inside. He rarely expressed his feelings. The two babies were as well behaved as one can expect of babies, but they required lots of care, time and affection, all of which seemed to be in short supply. I still was working at the Air Force Base as the Chief of Pediatric Hematology/ Oncology and they expected me to be there not only in body but in spirit as well.

My disbelief and anger about what had happened were immense and difficult to tolerate. I felt angry at Bella. I could not understand how she could have let this illness happen to her. I knew such feelings seemed irrational and selfish, but I could not figure out what had happened to my previously comfortable and predictable life. I was on a roller-coaster of painful emotions going up to highs that were artificially high when things seemed to be going well and unbearably low when Bella felt poorly or had to be in the hospital.

One night, about four months into the nightmare, I was driving her back to the hospital from a brief pass. I suddenly realized that *my anger had been misdirected*. The knowledge hit me just as if I had run face-first into a brick wall. I turned to Bella and blurted out, "You really don't want to be sick, do you?"

I really did not expect an answer, but I knew that I had experienced a major insight. Bella wanted her life back even more than I did. I suddenly realized that she was even more frightened, angry, depressed and miserable than I could ever be. I was no longer angry. Instead, I was filled with enormous sadness and pity. I spent the next several weeks getting to know, respect and love my sister-in-law in a way that I never had before. She relapsed for a third time in June. Her doctor offered her another course of chemotherapy and Bella considered going through treatment again. I knew that she would not survive a fourth treatment. Bella desperately wanted to live, but none of us ever did have control over what her leukemia was going to do. I told her that she should come home and spend time with her family who loved her rather than die in misery in the hospital. It was a very difficult and painful decision for her and for us.

Marian was the ultimate and consummate hospice nurse. Bella was weak, but Marian made sure that she had no pain. Knowing we would not have any more opportunities, one day we went to have a family portrait done. It took hours to get Bella ready. The bath wore her out so much that she had to rest for an hour before she could get dressed. Getting dressed wore her out again and it was another hour before her make-up could be applied. We arrived at the photographers in the middle of the afternoon for an appointment that had been scheduled for ten in the morning. The photographer was quite gracious about our tardiness. Bella looked wonderful. In the pictures that were taken that afternoon, the only one who was consistently smiling was Bella. Near the end of the sitting, Stephanie, who was now 8 months old, reached out for Bella's hair. We all got a good laugh thinking about the photographer's reaction if she had been able to pull her aunt's wig off her head.

Bella died just two days after the photographs were taken. She lapsed into a coma about 18 hours earlier. About one half-hour before she expired, only Marian was in the bedroom with her. Slowly, the entire family began to drift into the bedroom as if drawn there by some mysterious power. My niece said that she smelled roses and this bothered her because she was allergic to roses. She could not understand why anyone would have brought roses into the house. My mother-in-law also smelled the scent of roses. The aroma reminded her of her husband who used to bring her yellow roses every day as a symbol of his love. He had died several years earlier. The rose smell made my mother-in-law think that her husband had come to take his daughter home and had brought yellow roses with him. This was a very comforting thought. After we had all assembled in the room, Bella, who had not stirred for close to 18 hours, suddenly opened her eyes, looked at us with peace and warmth, and whispered, "I love you."

She then smiled, closed her eyes and stopped breathing. My niece let out an unearthly wail, "M-o-o-o-o-om" and started crying. With the realization that she truly had left us, we all began to cry. My babies did not understand what had happened—I wanted some time to grieve, but they still wanted to play. They did not need to be burdened with my adult concerns and so I put on their bathing suits and took them to the neighborhood pool. It was very strange sitting on the steps of the pool with my two daughters and wondering about the capriciousness and shortness of life. Because of her illness I had gotten to know Bella much better than if she had never had a cancer experience and we had both lived till we were 100 years old. I am very grateful for the time we spent together, but I still wish that we could have had just one more minute to spend together. But I know that if I were somehow granted that one minute, that I would then want one more and then another.

There is never enough time. Knowing these feelings from having lived them makes it easier to understand how the children I take care of and their parents feel. But it also sometimes makes it more difficult because I empathize with them so well.

Breaking Bad News

There are no classes that prepare a doctor on how to impart bad news. Only time and experience can give the doctor the needed empathy to transmit heartbreaking information in a sensitive and caring way.

I have learned a lot about various ways to talk with parents and children from my own personal experiences as well as from the reactions of patients and parents. When I learn of news that must be shared—news which I know will be difficult, I first make sure that I have all of the information I need to answer the difficult questions which are likely to follow.

Breaking bad news requires a direct person-to-person contact. It is important to give the news in person, not over a telephone or in a letter. Indirect methods may be easier for the bearer, but they are impersonal and cold. The news should be given in a comfortable and warm environment.

Sometimes it is necessary to speak to the parents with the children present. I feel that the child who is old enough and well enough to understand the information needs to be present. Under those circumstances, the discussions and breaking of the news may be done in the child's hospital room. I have found that the child not interested in hearing what I have to say will often fall asleep during the conversation. Sometimes I will have the initial conversation with the parents away from their child. That way, they can react to the shock and then gain some degree of composure before they return to their child's bedside.

Some teenagers, however, become suspicious of any discussions that are held with their parents but not directly with them as well. It is important to understand the family and their dynamics before proceeding. The doctor must take the individual family as well as cultural differences into account when discussing unhappy news. I try always to make sure that wherever such news is transmitted that everyone who is present has a chair to sit in and is comfortable before I proceed. The first time the difficult information is presented, I prefer that only the parents and the child be present. Later I will include relatives and friends in all other discussions if that is desirable to the parents.

I feel it is important that I be seated when giving bad news. I may be in a nearby chair or I may sit on the child's bedside (with the child's permission). I try to make strong eye contact with whomever I am sharing the news. If possible, I have some sort of physical contact as well.

Once the bad news is shared, the family usually retains little else of the conversation. The two things besides the news itself which I hope the family will remember are my caring, empathetic *attitude* and a sense of *hope*.

Some parents react to the news that their child has cancer with a blank stare and an empty, lost expression. Little information gets through at times like that, so I just try to find something positive to say. That way, if the parents recall anything of what I have just said, it will be something positive.

After a 24-hour period, most people have gathered themselves together enough to understand the facts about the disease and its treatment so that conversations and discussions can then be more focused and productive. Everyone reacts a little bit differently to the news that his or her child has cancer. Some sit in stunned silence while others cry. I have found that the reaction is related neither to the sex of the parent nor to their ethnic background. The image of the stoic father and the weeping, emotional mother is frequently wrong.

Some first impressions stick in my mind. When Chris was first diagnosed, he had been sick for 3 to 4 months. He had initially started to complain of headaches; his mother noted that he also had low-grade fevers. As time passed, the headaches became worse. He lost weight and continuously complained of body pains. His pediatrician at first was puzzled about the symptoms and instituted a series of tests to find their cause. The symptoms suggested that Chris had meningitis, an infection or inflammation of the lining of the brain. The pediatrician performed a spinal tap, a test to find out if meningitis was present. A spinal tap requires inserting a special needle into a space between the vertebral bones near the end of the spine and examining the clear fluid that is obtained. In Chris' case, the fluid which flowed out of the spinal needle was cloudy. The cloudiness was caused by large numbers of white cells that should normally not be found in spinal fluid. Various antibiotics and medications made no impact. An infectious disease expert and a neurologist lent their support to the pediatrician but to no avail. Chris continued to get worse. He lay curled in a fetal position, unable to sleep, eat or rest.

One day his pediatrician stopped me in the hallway and asked if I would take a look at the latest spinal fluid which had been obtained earlier that day. Four times over the previous two weeks, each subsequent spinal tap had been a bit cloudier and more filled with white cells than the last. I looked at the stained smear of the cloudy spinal fluid on a glass slide and saw malignant cells. I ordered special studies to be done on the spinal fluid that afternoon and they indicated that Chris had ALL.

ALL is a cancer of the white blood cells and is the most common cancer found in children. At one time, this type of leukemia was nearly always fatal, but, nowadays, nearly 75% of children with ALL can be cured. Chris' blood count, however, had no suggestion of the abnormalities that I had found in his spinal fluid. I obtained bone marrow from Chris' hip the next morning. This study confirmed that Chris had ALL. I was shocked when Chris' mother was delighted with the news. The knowledge that Chris had leukemia and that it could possibly be cured was far better information than what she had been receiving to that point. Not knowing what was causing her child's symptoms and watching him get progressively worse was much more agonizing than dealing with a diagnosis of leukemia. I had never before and have not since had a parent react with happiness to the diagnosis of ALL. In Chris' case it seems to have been appropriate. The fear of the unknown was more frightening and worse than a diagnosis of ALL.

A more stereotypical reaction to the diagnosis of malignancy was the way in which Ian's parents responded. Ian was a handsome young man of 11 years who was athletic and bright. One day he complained of feeling tired while playing soccer. A week earlier, one of his fellow team members had been diagnosed with infectious mononucleosis, and Ian thought he might have also contracted the disease. He was taken to his family physician for evaluation. His doctor was very surprised to find that Ian had an extremely elevated white blood cell count. The white count was so elevated that it represented a danger to the young man. Ian was admitted to the Pediatric Intensive Care Unit (PICU). I had never before admitted a patient to the PICU who just walked in and hopped up onto the bed. Perhaps I was just being cautious, but that white count sure scared me. After studies confirmed that Ian had Acute Myelogenous Leukemia (AML), I sat down with his mother and father to discuss the diagnosis and its treatment.

AML is similar to ALL in that both are cancers that arise from white blood cell precursors found in the bone marrow. However, the cells of origin are different. ALL is more common than AML in children and is more curable. However, recent treatments now allow nearly 50% of children diagnosed with AML to be cured. Ian's parents were aware that I suspected that their son had leukemia, but they were not prepared for me to verify that concern. The words, "I am sorry to tell you but your child has leukemia," were barely out of my mouth, when Ian's mother screamed and began to cry with huge, choking sobs. The boy's father bit his lower lip and tried to remain stoic.

His mother then began to shake her head rapidly back and forth and cry out, "Don't let my son die, Dr. Lazarus! Don't let my son die!"

Needless to say, we did not get much farther with discussions that evening. The next day, however, we were able to explore the options of therapy without a repeat of the earlier, passionate display. During the next two years, that mother became one of the strongest and most capable persons I have ever known. First impressions are not always correct. It is essential not only from a moral but also from a legal standpoint to inform parents of their child's disease, the planned treatment, the potential risks and benefits of that therapy, and alternatives to the planned treatment.

The notion that parents must be informed and must give consent to treatment (*informed consent*) before the therapy is undertaken arises from the basic belief that all humans have a right to self-determination. That means that each of us has the right to exercise some degree of control over what we will and will not allow to be done to our bodies. This concept is fairly straightforward when it applies to adults who are capable of making their own decisions. The idea of informed consent takes on a whole new meaning when it is applied to children. In the early days of treatment of childhood cancer, there was little that could be done for the child. Many textbooks from the 1950's and 1960's even suggest that it was unethical to disclose the diagnosis of cancer to a child because that knowledge would only serve to depress the child. As treatments became more successful and more children were cured of their cancers, the notion that children should be kept in the dark about their diseases while being forced to undergo intensive, painful and potentially dangerous treatments made less and less sense. Parents have both the right and the obligation to become informed about the nature of their child's illness and its treatment so they can make informed decisions about appropriate therapy.

Moral, ethical and practical issues raised by the concept of informed consent have become murkier. Questions include:

- Should have some role in making decisions about the treatment of their cancer.

- If so, at what age should they be given that role?

- Should parents be allowed to make decisions on a cultural or religious basis that may not seem to be the best choices for their children?

- If the guardians are not readily available, who should be allowed to make such decisions for minor children?

- What should be done, if anything, if parents refuse to allow their children to undergo a potentially life-saving treatment?

Dealing with children increases the questions. When I first meet and talk with parents after the child is diagnosed with some sort of cancer, they are almost always in shock and in denial.

The informed consent process involves going into detail about the nuances of complicated therapies. The nuances of such therapies are often so convoluted that even trained medical personnel have trouble following them. Yet we provide this very detailed information at a time when the parents are in an emotional state which is not conducive to the absorption of information. This has never seemed to me to be truly providing informed consent.

Shortly after a child has been diagnosed with cancer, I sit down and spend several hours with the parents to explain what is going on. The child, if old enough, is included in all of the discussions. I do not believe that most parents understand or appreciate much of what I tell them until many weeks, months or even years later. Much of the time I have the feeling that the families give consent for their child to participate in a treatment study because I subtly lead them to that conclusion. While I feel it is important for parents to be as informed as possible about the disease and the treatment, I am not convinced that informed consent as it currently is performed truly gives the parents self-determination.

There are no absolute best ways to tell a child that he or she has cancer. Much depends on the child's age. Children under the age of three have little, if any, concept of cancer. They are able to sense that something is terribly wrong and the tension they feel from their parents adds to any discomfort or pain they may feel because of the disease itself. I usually talk about the disease and the treatment in front of the child. I think it is important to make the treatment as matter-of-fact for the very young child as possible. We keep lots of toys and games in the outpatient area so the children can be distracted and can have fun even though they are getting chemotherapy. I know we have succeeded when a child cries because they do not want to leave after the day's treatment is completed.

Children acquire an ability to understand sickness and wellness somewhere around the time they are 5 or 6. The concepts they have are very concrete. I like to use the image that the cancer is like a bad army that has somehow invaded the child's body. I then use the image of the chemotherapy, surgery and radiation therapy as the good guys sent to fight back and win. Children who are less than 10 usually do very well with this concept and it is a fairly easy concept to explain. Some children will need more information about the specifics of their disease (such as where the cancer is, what its name is, the names of the specific medicines which will be used) while others do just great with the general concept.

Eric, for example, was 6 when he was diagnosed with ALL. After the diagnosis was confirmed, I sat down with his mother and father and spent about 3 hours reviewing the diagnosis and the plans for its treatment. I held the discussion at Eric's bedside. For most of the discussion Eric slept or watched television. Towards the end of my discussion, I asked Eric's mother and father if they would like to talk with Eric about why he was in the hospital and how he was going to be treated, or if they wanted me to discuss these issues with their boy. They both answered that they wanted me to tell Eric the news. Fortuitously, Eric awakened just as I finished asking the question. He did not wake up like I usually do. He had enjoyed a good nap and he felt rested. I looked at him and smiled.

"Eric," I said, "Do you know why you are here in the hospital?" The little boy said nothing. He just shook his head and kept his big brown eyes aimed at my face.

"Well, Eric," I continued, "your mom and dad brought you to the hospital and to me because you have a disease called leukemia. Do you know what leukemia is?"

Again the little boy shook his head. He looked briefly over at his mother and father and then focused his eyes on me again. "Let me try to explain what leukemia is. Leukemia is a disease that affects your white blood cells. Your white blood cells are cells that are found in your blood and they help your body fight off germs so that you stay healthy. Sometime ago, one of those white blood cells was attacked by an alien invader. You know, like in 'Star Wars.' Do you know what an alien is?"

Eric replied, "Is it like someone from outer space?"

I said, "It's exactly like someone from outer space only in leukemia the alien is much smaller so it can fit inside a white blood cell. Once it gets there, it changes the white blood cell so that it can no longer fight diseases. But this alien does something even worse. It gets that white blood cell to make many, many copies of itself. Soon there are so many copies of the bad cell that there isn't any room for all of the good cells. That's what happened to you. That alien attacked one of your white blood cells and turned it into a bad cell. Now your body is filled with those bad cells. That's why you haven't been feeling very good. Well, now we have a real tough job ahead. This alien doesn't want to leave your body. And if the alien does not leave your body, then you will not get well. We have a lot of armies that we plan to send into your body to help fight that bad alien. We can send them into your body through your mouth and through shots into your veins and your muscles. Now, I know that shots can hurt but it is the only way we can get the good armies into your body so that they can fight off this leukemia alien."

Eric was shaking his head, yes, but he had some tears in his eyes. I knew he was scared about the idea of getting shots even if that were the only way to fight off the alien army. "Eric," I said, "you and I are the generals of the good army. I make sure where and when the armies need to be put into your body. You are the general in charge of making sure that the armies have the best chance of working. You can do that by being strong and brave and trying to take your medicine whenever it is due to be given. Sometimes the good armies will make you feel kind of sick. You may get sick to your stomach or not feel real strong. Your hair may even fall out. But that is like what happens in a war. When two armies fight, the land and the people caught in the area where they are fighting sometimes get hurt too. But if we really work hard, we have a real good chance that we are going to get rid of that alien army. Eric, we are going to start the battle at 0800 tomorrow morning. Will you be ready to start the war?"

Eric nodded his head and I gave him a hug. "I look forward to working with you, General," I said. Eric just smiled and hugged me back.

The next morning when I came in at 8 a.m., Eric was bright-eyed and prepared. He had drawn a picture. It showed a boy in a bed. An IV line was attached to one arm. He had drawn pictures of a tank, an airplane, and a rifle in the air surrounding the little boy. "That's me," he said proudly pointing at the picture of the child, "I'm ready, Dr. Lazarus."

I don't believe that any other child I have cared for has ever bought the story as completely as Eric did.

Adolescents usually have a fairly adult ability to understand sophisticated concepts. Explaining to them the basic ideas about cancer and its therapy is not much different than explaining the same things to their parents. The problem is that adolescents also have difficulty accepting that something bad has happened to them because that means that they are not immortal. They also have to deal with the side effects of therapy and this can sometimes impact on their ability to make informed and rational decisions. Adolescents tend to be very present-oriented and have a great deal of difficulty looking at issues of delayed outcomes and consequences.

It is now a requirement that if the doctor and the parents feel that the child can understand the disease and its treatment, that they must give assent to the treatment. Minors cannot give consent. Assent means that they understand the information that has been presented to them and they agree to proceed with treatment. However, if an adolescent becomes distressed at the thought of losing his or her hair and refuses to give assent, the parents have the ultimate decision since they are the ones who are legally capable of giving formal consent. I find that it is actually easier to meet a new family and initially diagnose a cancer than to have to tell a family that their child's cancer has recurred. When I first meet a family, I don't know them and they don't know me. I don't know what to expect and I almost always have something positive to offer. So many children respond to therapy and so many of them are cured that the positives and excitement of beginning a new adventure often outweigh the horror of the diagnosis. But after knowing the family for a while, I become a part of their lives and they become part of mine. Saying, "I'm sorry," or "I have bad news" or some other statement does not work well when one knows the family well. The parents and the children have learned the nuances and realities of cancer well. They also know me all too well. They know when I am upset, sad, happy, excited or tired. I cannot hide my disappointment and sadness nor am I usually successful at making a relapse seem to have a positive side. While what news is given is of critical importance, the way that information is imparted is often even more so.

Usually only one parent comes into the office with the sick child during the course of his or her treatments. That parent may not be aware when I am concerned that the child has developed a new cancer or had a relapse of the old one. It is very important to have family support systems available at times like these, but there is no easy way to call other family members and apprise them of the situation without arousing undue feelings of alarm. If the missing parent or family member is at work and receives a message from the doctor that his or her presence is needed, most think only of horrible things that could be happening.

There is no way to lightly say, "Please come to my office for a discussion about your son's (or daughter's) illness."

At the same time, there is no adequate way to give bad news over the telephone. Alan's father told me later how he reacted when he received bad news about Alan while at work. Alan was 7 years old when he first presented with symptoms of acute leukemia. When seen by his pediatrician, Alan had an enlarged liver and spleen, swollen lymph nodes, and an elevated white blood cell count. ALL was the cause. After a thorough evaluation and discussion with both parents and the boy, we began therapy. Alan had an excellent initial response and was soon in remission. Many months later Alan came in for a routine monthly visit. His blood count showed that his white blood cells and platelets were unexpectedly much lower than anticipated. His chemotherapy was held and we waited for Alan's blood count to improve. Initially we thought that the decrease was due to an unusual reaction to the chemotherapy, but after two weeks with no chemotherapy, Alan's counts actually began to worsen a bit. I had warned Alan's parents that if the low blood counts persisted, I would need to look at his bone marrow to make sure that the bone marrow suppression was not due to the return of the leukemia. The day of the bone marrow examination, Alan and his mother came in alone. His father could not get away from work. The bone marrow studies showed what we all had feared the most. Alan's leukemia had returned. How was the news to be handled? Alan's mother tolerated things much better if her husband was at her side, but there was no good way to notify him at work without creating enormous fear. With great trepidation, I called Alan's father.

I gently said, "Jerry, is there any way you could come to my office now?"

His answer was an anguished, "You found something! What is it? Oh, my God!"

I simply replied, "Let's just talk about it when you get here." Jerry later told me that he had to get a co-worker to drive him to my office as he was so shaken by my call. The preparation for the news for both parents was nearly as bad as the news itself. When I later asked Alan's parents if there could have been a better way for me to have handled the situation, they both responded that they preferred to be together when such news was given. They said that I had handled the catastrophe as well as it could have been done. I still feel that there has to have been a better way.

I certainly know that the way in which I learned that I had a skin cancer was probably the worst way possible. I had gone to a dermatologist because I had a raised area on my forehead that would not go away. I had a biopsy done of the lesion during a quiet period just before lunch one day. Later that same afternoon I was talking with an 11-year old boy and his parents about his newly diagnosed brain tumor. I was well into my explanation of the disease and the proposed treatment when I received a page over my beeper. The message read, "Call Dr. So-and-so as soon as possible."

I stepped out of the boy's room and called. The dermatologist told me, "You have cancer. Come see me some time so we can talk about it." The juxtaposition of the way in which I was told about my skin cancer and the way in which I had notified the family that their child had a brain tumor was quite ironic. I felt betrayed by that dermatologist. When I went to his office later that day, he told me that he had seen thousands of skin cancers and that they were no big deal. I replied that I had seen only one and so my viewpoint of the importance of that skin lesion was far different from his. I knew that I was fair-skinned and that I was at risk for skin cancer, but there is a difference between knowing that it can happen and really having it happen. When I developed skin cancer at age 37, I felt that I was no longer immortal and my body would truly age. I was confused, angry and lost. I regained my equilibrium within a very short time but I realized that my idea of appropriate counseling and sensitivity to the feelings of patients with cancer did not extend to all doctors.

When I go to a doctor for a medical problem, I automatically assume that the doctor is knowledgeable, caring and bright. I think that most people make just such an assumption about their physician in order to establish a meaningful doctor-patient relationship. However, there are differences between physicians both as individuals and as caregivers. All doctors have to go through four years of medical school. In those four years they are expected to learn everything they can about an exponentially expanding amount of information about the human body and its function. Since the time I completed my training just a handful of years ago, even my subspecialized field has become further subdivided into smaller areas of study. Diseases have not changed to a great extent, but what is known about them has greatly expanded and evolved. In the quest to learn as much as possible about this ever enlarging base of knowledge, the human, caring and loving aspects of medicine have assumed a lesser role in the management of illnesses. There is little time for the medical student to learn the art of medicine in the four short years that are usually spent in medical school. Even during the years and the myriad of experiences that shape each of our lives which follow, the average doctor often continues to rely on technology to solve a patient's problems. Doctors come in all shapes, sizes, ability levels, colors and religions. Although all are (or should be) selected for their academic achievements in college, some are very good at memorization and still others are warm and caring but relatively poor at retaining facts. There are some who are very good with their hands and who have good hand-eye coordination and others who are nonathletic. Some doctors are in the profession to make money while others are completely altruistic and devoted to the service of others. There are special ones who have a warm, empathetic bedside manner who are also extremely knowledgeable and expert. How does one find these special doctors who have all the special qualities one would desire in a physician? There is no way to rank physicians or rate them once their schooling is finished. Even the standings in medical school do not take into account the ability to interact well with patients. The only way to find the physician who is right is to admit that doctors, like all people, are human and have some qualities which are good and some which are less so. Each person must determine those qualities that are important to him or herself. When he or she finds a physician who possesses those qualities, that person needs to be supportive and demonstrative of their gratitude. If the doctor they find does not meet his or her needs, he or she must be willing to ask for a second opinion or request a change. Complaining about that doctor will not change his or her behavior nor improve the doctor-patient relationship. The medical relationship goes both ways—from doctor to patient but also from patient to doctor. Those relationships work best in which all involved actively participate. When the doctor who diagnosed my skin cancer disappointed me, I chose to go to a different physician. This ability to choose is critical for both doctor and patient in order to be able to establish a successful doctor-patient relationship.

The danger of current attempts to alter the medical system in America is that such an alteration may diminish the patient's right to choose his or her own doctors. By so doing, this diminishes or even eliminates the responsibility that both the doctor and the patient have to ensure a mutually agreeable and respectful relationship.

Knowing what to do when someone is sick and knowing how to communicate that knowledge are two very different things. The ability of the medical professionals to extend themselves and provide love, support and empathy requires much more than knowledge. It requires a physician who truly embodies the art of medicine. Before the technological revolution of the last half of the twentieth century that brought many medical marvels, doctors had few sophisticated tools with which to work. However, the esteem and love in which they were held easily exceeds that of today.

Doctors were concerned with their patients. They treated them with respect. Physicians recognized that often there was little they could do except offer support and their presence and they gave of both freely. Dying was a fact of life, greeted with sadness but accepted for the natural process it was and remains. Children died more often in their early years than today. Few were the families that did not suffer the death of at least one child from some now preventable disease. The limitations of medicine and of doctors were accepted and accommodated.

Recently, I sat in the PICU with two of my colleagues, one a *pediatric intensivist* (a recently developed subspecialty of pediatrics which concerns itself with the care of children in intensive care units) and a *nephrologist* (a doctor who specializes in the care of kidney diseases). We were trying to figure out the best treatment to help a teenager who was suffering from liver failure. We talked about ways to remove toxins from her blood—toxins that would normally be removed by the young woman's diseased liver. As we reviewed several possibilities, discussing the benefits and risks of each, we came to realize how much the practice of medicine had changed since we left medical school. Although each of us was fairly young, we had all seen remarkable changes which had impacted, greatly on our practices. The nephrologist remembered how she had stirred dialysis powder in an open vat with a wooden paddle before using a cumbersome dialysis machine to remove waste products from people's bodies when their kidneys were unable to do it for them. All three of us had witnessed the onset of AIDS, Legionaire's Disease, central venous catheters, home health care, bone marrow transplants, magnetic resonance imaging (MRI) and computed tomography (CT), just to name a few of the amazing changes. We had also seen many new medications, routine organ transplants, new techniques in surgery which allow people to have organs removed and go back to work in one week with few ill effects. We were amazed how much had changed in such a short time and how much we now use which we take for granted.

What was once considered defensive medicine used to ward off lawyers or experimental medicine is now simply good care. Fantastic new ideas and techniques that were once the province of science fiction novels combined with a public media that has emphasized the positives and the successes of modern therapy without mentioning or glossing over the failures, side effects, and emotional and financial costs have led to a marked increase in the expectations of the general public. Even those who work well in the medical profession have heightened beliefs in the modern technologies. The belief that somehow all diseases are amenable to some sort of treatment combined with modern methods of medical financing have led to a more depersonalized system where the *art of caring* has become the *art of knowing which tests* and *which surgeries to use* rather than the *art of teaching families and patients how to cope better with illness*.

Miracles Happen

Many times when I meet someone new, especially someone not connected with the medical profession, they will ask me why I chose such a specialized field in which to practice. Most people feel that what I do and see each day must be very depressing. I have been told by other medical professionals who work in many different fields that I must be a special person because they could not stand to see a child suffer. That statement suggests that I must enjoy watching children suffer; nothing could be further from the truth. One of the reasons I love what I do is really quite simple. I feel that no other area of medicine allows a doctor, his or her patients, and their families to become as close or to share as deeply as the field of pediatric oncology does. Many people fear the intimate relationships and the total commitment it takes in order to provide good care.

With more and more children being cured of cancer each year, there are fewer sad days and difficult times. Even when a child dies, the knowledge that I may have helped that child depart this world with less pain and with dignity is very comforting. When I see that family recover from the pain of losing their child and watch them grow as individuals and as a unit, I know that what I have done is worthwhile.

Another reason I love what I do is that every now and then, miracles happen. I don't know why they happen or how to plan for them, but I do know they happen. I do not know if these miracles occur out of divine assistance or because of the sheer obstinacy of some children's spirits. I really didn't care when they occurred and I don't care now. All that I cared about was that the family's prayers and my prayers were answered.

What I consider a miracle is when a child with a very bad prognosis not only does not die but recovers. A child recovers from overwhelming odds. The first miracle occurred while I was in my training to become a pediatric oncologist. Samantha was 18 years old when I first met her. I had been away from the hospital for two weeks on a vacation and had just returned to work on the day she came into the hospital. Samantha had been a healthy, happy, slightly overweight farm girl when she got sick. She developed a fever and had finally gone to her local doctor when the fever continued even after a few days of home remedies. A blood count showed that all of her blood cells were reduced in number. Samantha had developed *aplastic anemia.*

Aplastic anemia is a medical condition where the bone marrow stops making blood cells. There are no abnormal or cancer cells involved, but the lack of normal cells has some profound consequences. Without enough white blood cells, red blood cells and platelets, the person develops fevers, infections, bleeding, weakness and fatigue. Without correction of the bone marrow problems, an overwhelming infection, internal bleeding or some other catastrophe will eventually result in the patient's death. While the cause of the bone marrow failure can be determined in some cases, in others the reasons for it are never determined. The local doctor reacted to Samantha's abnormal blood counts and quickly sent her to our hospital. Within a few hours of arriving and being assigned to a bed on the adolescent wing of the hospital, she needed to be transferred to the PICU. Samantha had developed pneumonia as a result of not having enough white blood cells. The bacteria causing the pneumonia found little resistance to spread. Within hours, the germs had entered Samantha's blood stream where they caused even greater havoc. The bacteria not only infected other organs, but they released toxins that further weakened already stressed internal body parts. Samantha's immune system reacted to the bacteria as well as it could. Substances were released into her blood stream to fight the bacteria, but these caused irritation and leaking of her blood vessels which further aggravated the dangerous situation. Samantha's heart could not keep up with the demands of her oxygen-starved body and fluid began to back up into her already diseased and congested lungs. Emergency medical procedures were instituted to try to support her overtaxed heart and lungs. The toxic chemicals released into the bloodstream set off a cascade of clotting proteins throughout the teenager's body. The excess coagulation initially affected the veins heading out of her liver. The clots in those veins produced blockage of the flow of blood from the lower half of her body as it traveled through the liver on its way back to the heart. The back-flow of blood that was now unable to pass through the liver caused her liver and the kidneys to fail. Despite massive support with medicines and machines, Samantha's kidneys stopped producing urine. Because of the excess clotting occurring all over her body, she soon ran out of clotting proteins and began to bleed from several sites. In the space of 48 hours, Samantha had gone from a reasonably healthy young lady to a critically ill person with nearly every organ system damaged or controlled in some way.

It was a difficult and trying time because of Samantha's severe deterioration. At the same time that we were trying to fight the bacteria, we were also trying to discover why her bone marrow had failed in the first place and how to make it better. Even though Samantha remained in a critical state, teetering between life and death, the pneumonia did not worsen and her heart slowly began to beat stronger. After two days the bacteria seemed to be coming under control. Because her kidneys were still not functioning, the decision was made to send her to the hospital next door to the Children's Hospital. That hospital was the only one nearby where kidney dialysis could be done.

The pediatric resident assigned to Samantha's case sat beside me and cried as we prepared for the child's transport to the new hospital.

"Why are you doing this?" she asked in great anguish. "Can't you let her die in peace with some dignity?"

"I don't know what will happen and I don't believe that she is ready to die," I replied with as much reason as I could muster. I, too, had some misgivings about going forward with a difficult and risky treatment like dialysis when Samantha was so critically ill. Still, without dialysis, she would surely die. Samantha's parents were not ready for her to die and definitely wished for us to proceed with the dialysis. Since Samantha was now in a different hospital, she was under the care of a different physician. I stayed in close contact with her and visited every day. For the first five days, nothing changed. She remained on a respirator unable to breathe on her own. Her lungs, liver and kidneys were slowly improving but the changes were small and not very visible to those sitting at her bedside.

On the sixth day a strange thing happened. Her blood cell counts began to improve. As the white cell count improved, so did her condition. Within two weeks her bone marrow had returned to normal. It took a third week for her lungs to improve enough for her to be removed from the respirator. Physical therapy was started to get her sore, stiff joints working again. Soon she was eating, talking, walking and happy. It took seven weeks for her recover enough to be discharged, but when she left the hospital, every body system was back in working order. I saw her as an outpatient one month later. Because of the respirator tube that had been in place in her throat for over six weeks, her voice was deep and gravelly. She had lost 25 pounds as a result of her ordeal, but this was the amount of weight that she had been trying, unsuccessfully, to lose in more conventional ways. Rather than being disappointed, she was quite satisfied with these two side effects of her therapy.

Before she left I asked Samantha if she remembered much of her brief but eventful encounter with the medical system. She replied that most of her experience was a blur. My comment was that it was lucky that she could not remember because I did not believe that the treatment that she had undergone would ever turn out to be a popular method of weight control. She laughed, gave me a hug and left. I presume that her life turned out well, but I do not know for sure since I have not heard from her since that time. I still think of her whenever I care for another critically ill child. I pray that this child will also turn out to be another miracle.

When we talk about miracles, we must realize that one of the greatest miracles is how modern medical technology has been able to find a way to cure some children of cancers that used to result in their deaths.

Cory represents one of the best examples of a child whose life was changed by the miracles of modern medicine. Every time I see him, I am reminded of why I practice in this field. Cory was eighteen months old when I was called by a pediatric gastroenterologist to see him. He was an adopted child. He had an older brother who was the natural son of the couple he knew as his mother and father. After several years of trying to have another child, his parents found out that they were unable to have more children. They spent months and thousands of dollars before Cory came into their lives. Cory was a beautiful child. He had blond hair and bright, shiny brown eyes that sparkled with life and with a devilment which only a toddler can display and still seem to be totally innocent. When I first walked into his hospital room, Cory was lying in a crib. He was sucking his thumb and looking at me quietly. I soon learned that he was only resting before he turned on full throttle. Cory had a swollen abdomen. His mother had taken him to a pediatrician. That doctor had noted the liver mass that was the source of the swelling. He had admitted the infant to the hospital and had asked a *gastroenterologist* (a doctor who specializes in stomach, bowel and liver problems) to examine the little boy. That doctor quickly called me when he suspected that the mass was due to a cancer.

The first test we ordered was a CT scan of his abdomen. Because of Cory's age, he needed sedation so he would be still while the CT scan was being done. Although the radiologist and a nurse stayed nearby to make sure that Cory was all right during the procedure, his mother also stayed in the CT room with him. A lead apron covered her chest and abdomen to protect her from any stray X-rays. While the CT examination was underway, a priest who served as a hospital chaplain happened to walk through the radiology department. The CT technician noticed the priest and thought that he might be able to comfort the anxious mother who was moment by moment becoming more aware that her child had some sort of cancer. The priest came in and said a few kind words to the mother before he left to attend to his original mission. Cory's mother had a different take on the priest's visit. She figured that the doctors had seen something on the X-rays. She decided that the priest's visit meant that Cory was going to die and that the priest had been called to pronounce last rites. By the time she got back to the pediatric floor, she was near hysterics. It took several hours of reassurance by the nurses to calm her down, but eventually she realized that the priest's visit had been merely a coincidence. Her confidence was short-lived.

Within a few hours later it was confirmed that her son's abdominal swelling was due to a malignant liver cancer known as a *hepatoblastoma*. The gastroenterologist told her that he had never seen a child survive that kind of cancer. I gave the family a different prognosis.

Hepatoblastoma is a primary cancer of the liver that occurs most often in young children. It is a very rare cancer, its cause unknown, but it is not related to prior liver infections or to the foods the child has eaten. If the tumor can be removed surgically, it is often cured.

Many children with this tumor, however, have tumors too large to be removed when they are first diagnosed. Some of the hepatoblastomas have even spread to other organs like the lungs when they are first found. Cory's tumor involved both halves of his liver and could not be removed. As a result, surgery was not initially an option. Cory was started on a combination of chemotherapy drugs that had been shown in a small number of children who had hepatoblastomas to produce good responses. With the first round of the strong medications, Cory's abdomen began to shrink. The first course of chemotherapy was given in the hospital, but the treatment was very difficult on Cory and his mother. Cory hated not being active and his movements were restricted in the hospital.

Although we had never treated this type of cancer as an outpatient before, we decided to try in order to make life better for this child and his family. Despite the treatments, Cory did not slow down. He was like a tornado. As soon as he would enter my office, he would go into action. It would take him less than two minutes to have every toy and game strewn around the reception room floor. All the while, he would be smiling broadly even as he looked for something else to get into. Marian used to say that his mother gave him amphetamines before he came into the office. I just was glad that I did not have to take care of him at his home. I did not have the energy. The first course in the office was interesting. We did not realize that *extension tubing* should be added to the IV in order to give this miniature whirling dervish more slack. Before the chemotherapy was started, he needed to receive fluids through the IV to increase his flow of urine so that the medications could be given safely.

On the day he was due to start, Cory came into the office and was quickly ushered into a treatment room. There the IV was started. As soon as he could, Cory was up and running. The treatment room was linoleum covered and was about 20 feet away from the reception area. The reception area was carpeted. From the treatment room to the reception area was a step over a small rise since the carpeting was set higher than the linoleum. Cory negotiated this tiny rise with ease, but his IV, which was attached to a pole on wheels, was momentarily held up by the elevation. Cory did not stop but the IV did. The IV pole, which was attached to the short IV tubing which was connected to the catheter which ran inside Cory's vein, began to fall forward. Cory's mother dived for the pole. Other children and parents sitting in the reception area gasped as I also dived for the falling IV pole. I caught it just before it hit the ground. The excitement barely slowed the child, but he paused momentarily. This was long enough for his mother to gather him up and save him from a major disaster. Cory gave no sign that anything untoward had happened. He smiled his usual winning smile and began chattering in that gibberish that toddler's use which sounds like real talk but is not. His mother sighed deeply and, in all seriousness, asked what we could do to sedate her child. The medicine we were giving him to keep him from getting sick from the chemotherapy did make him sleepy, but it needed to be given just before the chemotherapy was started. The IV had to have been running for at least two hours before the chemotherapy was started. Therefore, his mother and I needed to make it through more than two hours of Cory's incredible energy before he could finally be given the *antiemetic* that caused him to sleep. By the time he fell asleep, all of us were worn out as well.

Hepatoblastomas often produce a substance, *alpha-fetoprotein*, which is a marker found in the blood for the amount and extent of disease that is in the patient's liver. Cory's alpha-fetoprotein, like virtually all children with hepatoblastomas, had been very elevated when he first started therapy. After the third course it reached a near normal value. Just before the fourth course was due to begin, the value started to rise a little bit. Cory was given the chemotherapy despite this slight increase in the value of the marker. A CT scan done the same day as the tumor marker was obtained had shown that the tumor was continuing to shrink. Because of the CT scan results, I was not too alarmed by the changes in the alpha-fetoprotein value. One week later, I repeated the alpha-fetoprotein level and the value was higher still.

I called a pediatric surgeon and told him that the time had come to remove the tumor. The surgeon was not very optimistic but it was either remove the tumor at that point or help the parents cope with the death of their adopted child. The Tuesday that Cory went to surgery was a day filled with tension. The surgeon told me that he expected the surgery to take between 6 and 7 hours. I was very surprised and disappointed when the child and the surgeon appeared in the PICU (Pediatric Intensive Care Unit) just four hours later. I was even more surprised, although very pleased, when the surgeon told me that he had been able to remove the entire tumor. He had found it to be an easier procedure than he had initially thought it would be. Cory is now eight years old. He is only a bit less active than when I first met him. I do not get to see him much anymore but that is because his family moved a few years ago. Every now and then his parents will call and let me know of his latest accomplishments and adventures.

I received another miracle in the mail just the other day. It was not the miracle itself, but an invitation to a birthday party for the miracle child. Little Eve was not supposed to be celebrating a second birthday, let alone her first birthday, but there was an invitation to her second birthday party sitting in my mailbox. I tore open the envelope and looked at the card that had been cut to look like a popular children's television character. I just smiled when I saw whom it was from. I thought about what this child had gone through just to be able to enjoy her second birthday. I had first learned about Eve on a Thursday afternoon about 20 months earlier. I had been running errands with my children when my beeper went off. It was a call from a local pediatrician. This doctor wanted me to know about a child whom I would be seeing the next day. He told me that Eve was just 7 months old but she appeared to have leukemia. He said that she had been having multiple problems for a few days and had come to see him. He had obtained a blood count because he thought that Eve looked pale. The blood count was very abnormal. The results of the test had not returned before the family had left to go home. Home was in a rural area quite a ways from the hospital and so he thought that she could wait 24 hours before being seen. The next day Eve and her parents were sitting in a treatment room in my office. She was very sick-appearing and I knew that this was going to be a problem.

Acute leukemia in infants is rare but is associated with a very poor outcome. The babies tend to respond poorly and relapse early even when they do respond. I was as positive as I could be with the two frightened parents trying to prepare them for what lay ahead. Eve was admitted to the hospital for further evaluation and treatment. Just starting an IV was a nightmare. Her veins were tiny. Just as soon as they were successfully entered, they would quickly collapse and blood would leak into her skin tissues. Finally, a tiny and tenuous IV line was placed and the necessary studies were obtained. We soon found that Eve had a leukemia that was a mixture of acute lymphocytic and acute myelogenous leukemias. A more permanent central venous catheter was placed the next day. Chemotherapy was then started.

Despite the initial dismal prognosis, Eve's leukemia cells began to quickly die from the effects of the powerful chemotherapy medications. She began to feel better. I still knew that her chances were poor, but hope can be a powerful sustainer. Her response and her happy behavior allowed us all to begin to hope just a little bit more. After two weeks she was well enough to leave the hospital and treatment continued as an outpatient. Four months passed and Eve continued to do well.

When she came in one day to receive some chemotherapy, she was feeling well and very happy. Unexpectedly, the microscopic examination of her blood cells showed the same changes that had been present when she had first been diagnosed. It was clear that the leukemia had returned. Eve's parents and I were devastated. No matter how aware of the prognosis one is and how realistically one faces the facts, the reality of a recurrence is a terribly difficult event. We discussed a new treatment and started a new chemotherapy program the very next day. The leukemia cells again responded and soon Eve's bone marrow looked clear of leukemia cells. Because of the powerful medicines the infant had received, there were few normal cells there either. Because her bone marrow lacked the normal cells she normally would have had in order to fight infections, she developed high fevers, mouth sores, and severe diarrhea. She was sicker than she had been when she had the leukemia cells and her parents began to wonder whether they had made the right decision to have their child receive a second round of chemotherapy. Slowly, though, Eve improved.

After a few more weeks, she began to behave with the same vigor and animation that had earlier made her a favorite of the pediatric nurses. Since the leukemia had returned so swiftly, we knew that Eve's only chance of survival was to undergo a bone marrow transplant. Even this offered only a minimal possibility of success because her initial relapse had occurred so quickly. A bone marrow transplant could only be done an alternative bone marrow could be found. Eve's sister did not match her and there was not enough time to look for a match in the National Marrow Donor Registry.

The National Marrow Donor Registry is a list of millions of people who have volunteered to donate their bone marrow to someone who may not be related to them, but who matches them anyway. The only decent remaining option was to use the mismatched marrow of her father, but this was fraught with all kinds of potential problems. I called a bone marrow transplant specialist in another state. This particular specialist had a lot of experience with the kind of transplant that I thought represented Eve's only decent hope. Fortunately, this bone marrow transplant specialist agreed to take the child as a patient.

Within a few days the details were worked out and Eve was on a plane to a state thousands of miles away. The departure was filled with anxiety and hopeful expectations. As Eve's parents and I hugged and said our good-byes, none of us knew whether we would see Eve come home alive again. It was now wintertime. In Texas it gets cooler at this time of year, but rarely cool enough to wear anything heavier than a sweater. Winter is something one reads about in books. Snow has fallen on this city only twice in the past 15 years. I do not think that Eve's family was quite prepared for the climate shock that greeted them. Fortunately, most of their time was spent indoors. Eve tolerated the chemotherapy and radiation given for the bone marrow transplant even better than she had the previous chemotherapy course. By March she was recovering well and preparing to return home.

As a precaution a bone marrow study was performed a few days before she was to leave. The studies of the bone marrow suggested that about 10% of her bone marrow cells were leukemic. It was clear that the leukemia was again returning. The feelings of despair and hopelessness were almost palpable through the phone wires when Eve's mother called to tell me the bad news and get some advice on what to do next. The options were now extremely limited. I knew that virtually no one who had relapsed following a bone marrow transplant ever survived. I had few ideas other than for the family to come home and prepare for the inevitable advance of the disease. The transplant doctor, however, had one further idea for treatment. He suggested that some of Eve's father's lymphocytes be gathered and then injected into Eve's system. The lymphocytes are the white blood cells that not only help fight infection but are also responsible for rejection of transplanted tissues. The hope was that her father's lymphocytes would reject Eve's leukemia cells. The idea had not met with great success on the few times it had been tried before on similar patients. Still, it was all that was left and it was worth a shot.

Shortly after receiving her father's lymphocytes, Eve became sicker than she ever had from any of the previous therapies that had been tried. Her skin turned bright red from a dense, total-body rash. She developed virtually uncontrollable diarrhea. More than once I was called by the transplant doctor because he was sure that she would not survive until the next day. He would then call the next day to say that somehow she had made it through the night. This went on for a few weeks until the calls began to come less and less often. Slowly, Eve improved and her abdomen and skin began to heal. The process was very slow and tedious but always in a positive direction. Finally, after more than 5 months, Eve was truly ready to come home. Even more remarkable, her bone marrow no longer showed signs of leukemia. The course since then has been filled with peaks and valleys. Eve is still seen in my office frequently but has only rarely been in the hospital. Each time she needs to receive a little less medicine and does just a little bit better. Her skin has nearly completely healed and her diarrhea has disappeared. She has grown slowly because of all the medicines she has been taking, but even that problem has improved in the past few months. Despite her short stature she has had fairly normal development. She is a full-fledged two-year old with a good command of the word, "No!"

Her birthday this year is truly a miracle. I hope there are many more to come.

Although Benjamin Kenneth (B.K. to his friends) does not represent quite the miracle experienced by Samantha, Cory or Eve, he definitely remains my miracle child. Few of the young persons I have dealt with since I entered this field have impacted or changed my life as much as B.K.

B.K., with behavior changes and headaches for a few months, began having difficulty with his vision, so a CT scan was done of his brain. This showed a large tumor, a *medulloblastoma*, growing in his cerebellum. The cerebellum is that portion of the brain that controls balance and fine motor movements. People with tumors in this region develop balance problems due to the tumor as well as severe headaches and vomiting because the medulloblastoma often obstructs the flow of the cerebrospinal fluid that circulates inside the brain. In B.K.'s case some of the cells from his medulloblastoma had spread throughout the fluid-filled spaces of his brain. Tumor cells had traveled to several other sites within the young man's brain. Once they settled there, they started to grow. Further X-ray studies showed that the medulloblastoma had spread throughout much of B.K.'s brain and spinal canal. His vision difficulties had been caused by the cancer cells growing in the area where the optic nerves meet inside the brain. After meeting with B.K.'s parents to describe the problem and the plans for treatment of this widespread malignancy, I went back to my office with the thought that I would start B.K.'s treatment the next day. However, when I came into the intensive care unit the next afternoon, I was surprised to find B.K. with a tube in his throat that was attached to a respirator.

He had seemed to be recovering well from surgery to remove the primary cerebellar tumor just the day before. When I walked onto the unit, his mother rushed up to greet me and asked, "What is going on?"

Since I had no idea myself, I told her that I would find out and let her know as soon as I could. It turned out that B.K. had suffered a seizure the evening before and had stopped breathing for a short time. The doctors who had been present at the time had to perform cardiopulmonary resuscitation (CPR) to save his life. He had been placed on medications to prevent further seizures. The medications as well as the seizure itself had rendered him totally unresponsive and dependent on the respirator to breathe.

B.K. the day before had not been talking but at least he could look around and show some sign that there was a person inside the physical shell. But when I walked onto the floor that day, it appeared that he was alive only because machines were doing all the work for him. At that time, and even today, a combination of radiation therapy and chemotherapy has resulted in very good outcomes for children with this type of brain tumor—if the tumor has not spread from the cerebellum when first diagnosed.

The children like B.K. whose tumors had spread wildly at diagnosis do not have as favorable an outcome, but even some of them can be cured. B.K. was in no condition to go to radiation and so the plan was to start chemotherapy first. B.K. was quite ill when the chemotherapy was started. It was hard to imagine that the chemotherapy could make him even sicker, but it did. The more we worked to correct the problems produced by the chemotherapy, the more other problems developed.

B.K.'s parents became more despondent with each passing day. They began to wonder why they had ever agreed to have B.K. receive chemotherapy. Finally, after 3 days of agonizing, they requested that no new therapy be instituted and that we try to withdraw as much as possible in order that they could take him home to die. It took about 10 more days to make all the necessary arrangements. B.K. no longer required a respirator, but he was unable to react to visual, tactile or auditory stimulation. He could not eat on his own so he was fed through a tube that led from his nose to his stomach (an NG tube). A hospice program was called so the family would have access to nursing and supportive care.

Several times each week a hospice nurse would go to B.K.'s home to see how the boy was progressing and to help the family care for their severely disabled boy. Once a week the nurse would call me and give me an update. As time passed and days became weeks and weeks became months, it became clear that B.K. was getting better. He still was not eating and could not move his legs, but he had begun to move his arms. He had also developed rudimentary communication skills. A salute or a wave of his hand indicated a positive statement while the raising of his middle finger was a symbol of frustration. It seemed strange for that particular gesture to be one of the B.K.'s first functions to return. After 4 months in hospice care, I finally caught on. B.K. was truly improving. I arranged for him to be admitted to the hospital for a full re-evaluation. My impression that B.K. had greatly improved was confirmed by my face-to-face examination and by the X-rays. The various brain abnormalities had decreased in size by at least half. I arranged for B.K. to be transferred to a rehabilitation hospital where he could receive intensive therapy to improve his muscle strength and motor movements and to teach him how to communicate once again. He also underwent the radiation therapy that had not been able to be given several months earlier.

B.K.'s parents registered their son with the Make-A-Wish Foundation while he was undergoing therapy at the rehabilitation hospital. Make-A-Wish is one of several such organizations in this country designed to grant the wish to a child with a life-threatening illness. Many of these groups suggest that the children need to be terminally ill when they are enrolled. Since I have never been able to predict who will live and who will die (and have no desire to try to do so) and I do not like the implications of signing a child up for such a program only if they are terminally ill, I use the term life-threatening illness. I think that it is important to maintain hope and to have something positive for the child and the family to enjoy which is entirely non-medical. Most of the children choose a trip to one of the large theme parks as their wish, but not B.K. Somehow, with a combination of salutes, waves, and middle fingers, he managed to let his family know that he wished to receive a signed baseball from the New York Mets. Shortly after his wish was communicated to the baseball team, a New York Mets' baseball cap and autographed baseball arrived in the mail. A day later B.K. received a call at the rehabilitation hospital from one of the Mets' players. The scene in the room was electrifying. Half of the nursing staff as well as doctors and his family stood at the door to his room while B.K. lay with the telephone held to his ear and listened. B.K. excitedly waved his arms, smiled and raised his middle finger in response to the voice on the other end of the line. After about 15 minutes, the phone call ended. As the receiver was placed back in its cradle, B.K. looked up and in a very rusty, quavering voice called out, "M-O-M". This was the first word his mother had heard B.K. speak in over 6 months. She started crying with tears of joy.

I do not know if that baseball player who has since retired ever learned what an impact he made on a young man who was desperately ill. Rehabilitation was not easy. Almost 6 months of not moving and not speaking required a lot of hard work to overcome. B.K. stayed in the rehabilitation hospital for almost two months before he was able to graduate to an outpatient therapy program. At first when he left the hospital and needed to come into the office, he would arrive in a wheelchair. He could not sit up completely in the chair. Slowly over the next few weeks, he learned to sit up and even to stand again. It was a special and exciting day when he took his first step in almost one year. After several months the wheelchair was returned to the American Cancer Society because he no longer needed it. Speech returned even slower. The call from the baseball player had been the catalyst, but at first he was only able to say a few words. Unfortunately, much like the hand gestures, the first words that returned were curse words. B.K. had absolutely no idea of the impact of these words and said them in the same manner that someone might say, "Please" or "Thank you." Sometimes it was difficult not to laugh.

B.K.'s speech pattern had a peculiar rhythm to it. There was little inflection to his voice and each syllable and word received the same emphasis. After a nurse did something for him, he would say in his unusual singsong pattern, "Thank you, bitch." The nurses were quick to remind B.K. of the appropriate terms, but they never were offended by his comments since they were never meant to offend. The reaction of those that first met B.K. and did not know of his proclivity to use such vulgar vernacular was often quite humorous.

Because his tumor had grown near where the optic nerve entered into the brain, B.K. was blind. This inhibited his rehabilitation to a great extent because it took years for him to accept this disability. Only recently has he worked to learn Braille. Once he got well enough, he returned to school. While there were definite deficits now present in his learning abilities, B.K. had retained an excellent memory. He was able to keep up in school in several subjects but not all. The schools, however, were not prepared for B.K. Schooling for children with learning disabilities in only a few areas like B.K. can be limited and limiting. Most public schools have programs for children with severe disabilities, but there are few opportunities for children whose learning disabilities are severe in only a few areas.

I have come to rely heavily on a neuropsychologist to find the specific defects in learning which uniquely affect each such child. A neuropsychologist is person who has a graduate degree in psychology and who specializes in understanding and improving the development and education of children. Such a professional may also work with adults who have sustained various kinds of brain damage. The neuropsychologist with whom I work spends several hours with the child. After extensive testing and evaluation of the child, the neuropsychologist will then work with that child's school to develop an individualized and appropriate program. Some children have tremendous potential as long as they do not have to do any problem solving. Others have difficulty if the lessons are presented verbally, but do great if they are visual. Each child must be treated on an individual basis and have a learning program created unique for his or her problems.

Despite our best efforts, B.K. was placed in a class for severely disabled children. Most of the workers in the class served as caretakers for the children. Teaching and learning were not their main goals. B.K. felt insulted and angry. His blindness only increased his frustration. He would act out in class and use his profane vocabulary with impunity. This got him in constant trouble. The schools were not as easygoing about B.K.'s vocabulary as the hospitals were. One day Marian asked B.K. why he did not listen at school and why he cursed at the teacher when he never did that to us when he was in our office. B.K. answered that it was because we always treated him with respect. We knew he could understand and that he had opinions that mattered. Once we worked with him to express his concerns at school in an appropriate manner and got the teachers there to understand how to listen, the problem improved. B.K.'s use of vulgar language lasted a long time but has now essentially disappeared.

The neuropsychologist once asked B.K. whether he had ever been a member of the Boy Scouts. B.K. answered in his sincere monotone, "Oh yes, doctor. I used to belong to the Boy Scouts, but I had to quit. Those fuckers use bad language." The neuropsychologist had to bite his lip to keep from laughing.

Once he had himself under control, the neuropsychologist replied, "That certainly is a good reason not to be a member of such an organization."

B.K. is Hispanic but he has very light-colored skin. His ethnic heritage gives him great pride. One time he came into my office and I asked him what he had been doing the previous week. He said he had been to see the neuropsychologist. I asked, "Did you have a good time, B.K.?"

"Oh yes, Dr. Lazarus," answered B.K. "That doctor is my favorite white doctor."

"But B.K.," I exclaimed with mock sadness, "how could you like him more than you like me?"

"I'm sorry, Dr. Lazarus," was his reply. "You definitely are my favorite white doctor."

I am proud to state that I still retain that status. B.K. is an appreciator of people and of life. One day he said, "Miss Marian, you are so beautiful." Then he granted her one of his brightest smiles.

She said, "Thank you very much, B.K., but how can you tell that I am beautiful. You can't see me."

" But, miss, you always smell so beautiful that I know that you must be beautiful." Later he told her that he wanted to marry her because she was so good to him. Several weeks later he said that he no longer wanted to marry Marian because he wanted to marry me. His mother said, "But, B.K., you are not gay."

He answered, "Neither is Dr. Lazarus."

Marian then asked, "Well, why do you want to marry him?" His response was quite insightful. "Miss, I have had cancer for several years now and in that time, I have had 14 different doctors. None have been as good to me as Dr. Lazarus. I know that if I were married to Dr. Lazarus, he would always be good to me and I would have a wonderful life."

It has been a wonderful honor and privilege to help B.K. About three years after he first went home to die because he was so ill, the tumor recurred. B.K. had to start back on chemotherapy. Instead of being a difficult problem, it enabled me to see him more often. I loved it when he would come in because I knew that there would always be a big smile and a deep laugh that came from deep within his soul. Recently he was in the hospital for a course of chemotherapy. He had a roommate who was his age and who also was my patient. The two of them hit it off well. When I came in on rounds to see them, B.K. was in the bathroom with the door closed. I said hello to his mother and to his roommate and said I would be back later to examine B.K.

Suddenly a voice came out of the bathroom, "Hello, Dr. Lazarus."

I replied, "I hear a voice but I don't see the body to which it is attached. It must be God. Hello, God. What can I do for you?"

B.K.'s voice continued, "Is my roommate going home tomorrow?"

My answer was, "I certainly hope so, God, but I am not sure. But since you know everything, God, you already know the answer. Tell me, is your roommate going home tomorrow?"

By now B.K.'s roommate and his mother were smiling broadly at the exchange. B.K.'s answer did not disappoint them. "I'll leave that up to you. By the way, go to church," he said. With that, we all began to laugh.

More than 7 years have passed since B.K. first entered my life. Once again his tumor is growing. This time I think that the medulloblastoma will finally accomplish what it nearly did so long ago. No matter when B.K. dies, he will always be my miracle child.

Quality of Life

When I started my training, there were no *central lines*. A central line is a tube placed into a major vein that functions as a means of access into a patient's circulatory system. The tube is placed into the vein by a surgeon and then threaded to a point near the heart. The other end of the tube is then tunneled under the skin so that it exits the body some distance away from where it enters the vein. A central line allows easy access to the blood system. Initially, when first used in Seattle in the late 1970's, these central lines (or central venous catheters) were used for feeding someone intravenously when their throat or stomach or intestines did not work right. The value of these central venous catheters was quickly recognized. Soon, central lines were being used for drawing blood, giving medicines and all sorts of other uses that required access to the venous system.

These central lines have been a wonderful advance and have reduced pain and suffering for many children and adults. Giving chemotherapy requires frequent and accurate entry into the vascular system. During my training before there were central venous catheters, I remember putting IV's into tiny thumb veins in the middle of the night so that chemotherapy could be given or continued when the original IV came out. I remember children with burns in their skin because the chemotherapy had leaked out of their veins into the surrounding tissues. Even when the chemotherapy managed to stay in the veins, the children were miserable because of all the painful needle sticks required to get a decent IV started. After a while their veins would become scarred and brittle and almost impossible to hit accurately. The children were often afraid of the doctors and nurses. With the central lines, they no longer need to be fearful.

Many years ago while learning the art of pediatric oncology, I was the doctor for a handsome two-year old boy who had a tumor growing in the right side of his face just below his eye. For five straight days every four weeks for two year, she received chemotherapy. Each month, at the start of treatment, his mother would bring him to the clinic so he could have an IV placed in one of the tiny veins on the back of his hands. He was an amazingly cooperative young man who would sit quietly in his mother's lap while a doctor or nurse explored his hand searching for a usable vein. Over time the veins became more and more elusive. He rarely cried. One Monday I was the person expected to start his IV. Just as the needle found its target, he reflexively pulled his hand away and the needle missed. He looked at me in amazement, pain and fear and then started to cry.

Through his tears he sobbed, "I Sorry!" I reached over and hugged him.

"No," I answered, "I am sorry. I am so sorry that I have hurt you and I am even sorrier that I have made you feel responsible. I am so sorry that I hurt you."

That little boy has now grown into a terrific teenager, but he still remembers his treatments only because he remembers how much he hated having the IV's placed. Central lines have ended such memories. When central lines were first introduced, the only types which were available were those that exited the skin to the outside. These types require a fair amount of care in order to remain functional and disease-free.

A short while after these kinds of lines were introduced, a second kind was developed. The newer kind of central catheter has a port or a reservoir at the end of the tube that normally exits the skin. The port is made of a special plastic that is held in place by a metallic holder. This port remains under the skin. The port is accessed with a special needle. Children with this kind of catheter still have to have a shot, but the injection is much quicker, easier and less painful than trying to find a small vein in the hand. Although I know that central lines are one of the changes that have made cancer therapy better, I know that if they were so wonderful, we would all have one placed right after birth. That way, none of us would ever have to worry about being stuck or having IV's. Each particular type of catheter (and there are now several) has its own distinct advantages and disadvantages. It is unusual when dealing with a young child with cancer for the disadvantages to outweigh the advantages. Many of the cancer treatments now given even require that a catheter be placed because of the way in which the chemotherapy will be given. These catheters have made new therapy techniques feasible and have also made the lives of these children much better. Still, we must never take these catheters for granted since they can produce an increased risk of infection and clotting.

At first, the only children who had a catheter placed were those in whom all means of access into their veins had been exhausted. After I left my training program to enter the Air Force, I rethought the use of these catheters. It seemed to me that central lines had been developed to improve the quality of life for children with cancer. It made no sense to give chemotherapy, and then, when the veins were no longer patent, to put in the catheter. If the catheter was good enough to be used after the regular veins were no longer patent, then it was good enough to be used at the beginning of therapy when the veins were still intact. My feelings about the catheters were obviously shared by many other pediatric oncologists because there are now very few children who do not have a central line placed at the time they are diagnosed with cancer.

Several years ago I sent a patient with an abdominal tumor to a very aggressive pediatric surgeon. The surgeon placed a central venous catheter in the child at the same time he removed the tumor from his abdomen even though he did not know what kind of tumor had been removed. I admired the surgeon's progressive attitude and his enthusiasm even though that child ended up not needing the catheter. The surgery alone had cured the tumor. It takes a lot of work by the parents to keep the central lines that exit the skin clean, unclotted and uninfected. Good education and patience are needed to teach the families the proper technique and to follow up to make sure that certain standards of care are met. These lines make swimming, bathing and some other activities more difficult. They may affect the body image of older children and adults. Despite all these potential problems, these lines are great. The age of the child may affect the choice of the type of central venous catheter that is selected. Still, some very young children have been able to use the variety of central venous catheter that exits the body despite the many potential and real problems associated with them. Most of these children do not play with their catheters and often even participate in their care. They may even treat the catheter as part of their body if they are left in long enough.

Henry had his catheter placed when he was four months old so he could receive treatment for a malignant tumor arising from his prostate gland. He received chemotherapy on a regular basis for two years and his parents did a terrific job caring for the catheter. It was always clean and uninfected. Henry never played with the catheter even as he grew old enough to get into everything just like every other toddler. When the chemotherapy ended and the time came to remove the catheter, Henry became very upset because the surgeon removed the catheter and did not give it back to him to keep. That catheter was like an arm or a leg would be to us. It was much more to him than just a tube through which blood was drawn and chemotherapy was given.

April regarded her catheter as something that served as a rite of passage. She was diagnosed at age three with ALL and her catheter had been placed so she could receive treatment. She was not only puzzled but also angry that her younger brother did not have a catheter placed when he turned three. In her mind, the only reason that she had had the catheter was because she had turned three. April had convinced her brother that he would get his catheter around the time he reached the age of three. It took his mother and me nearly two weeks to convince the little boy that he did not really need a central line. Now that April is a teenager, she still wishes that her brother would have surgery, but I think now her reasons are different.

Although many toddlers do not play with their central venous catheters, some young children have an insatiable curiosity and a need to investigate and explore everything. A catheter sticking out of the chest is a wonderful temptation. George and Jack were both little boys with ALL. George was just two years old while Jack was nearly four. Both showed us that we needed to be prepared for every eventuality when it came to children with catheters. George was in the hospital for chemotherapy when someone accidentally left a pair of scissors on a table beside his crib. George often watched as his mother and the nurses would clamp the catheter whenever they were working on it. The clamp that was used closely resembled a pair of scissors. The major difference, of course, was that the clamp did not have any cutting edges. George, like the namesake monkey, was curious to try such a new item. He reached for the scissors. Before anyone realized what he was doing, he took a healthy slice through the line. Blood poured out of the tube since the blood was now free to flow with none of the usual hindrances that should be present at the end of a catheter. George's mother had been sitting at the toddler's bedside while he performed his handiwork. Fortunately, she quickly noticed the mess, and the chaos that erupted was relatively brief. I am sure to his mother that it seemed like the bleeding went on for a long time, but once she realized why her son had suddenly begun to bleed from his chest, she grabbed the correct clamp and the blood flow was quickly stopped. Fortunately, George had cut his catheter at a point that allowed it to be easily repaired. About an hour later, still unnerved by her harrowing experience, George's mother called Marian to tell her what had happened.

Marian's response was unexpected. She exclaimed, "Isn't that wonderful?" as if she had just been told that George had won the Nobel Prize.

"Isn't that wonderful?" screamed George's mother in disbelief, "He could have bled to death."

"Oh, I know. That must have been just horrible. But isn't it wonderful that George, who is only two years old, has the dexterity to use scissors. There are not many children I know who are that talented." Somehow, Marian is always able to see a positive side to every situation.

Jack was a few years older than George was but he also managed to do exactly the same thing to his catheter. This time the child's experimentation with scissors occurred at home. Once again, the child's mother was right there to put the correct clamp on the catheter and stop the flow of blood before disaster occurred. Shortly after Jack performed his catheter surgery, his mother called me in a panic. I told her to bring the boy to the emergency room right away. In those days there were no specialized nurses who were trained to patch broken catheters. As a result the surgeon who placed the catheter was responsible for any necessary repairs. I arranged for that surgeon to meet me at the emergency room so we could jump into action as soon as Jack arrived. Both the surgeon and I were new in practice and relatively naive. We wanted to be known as physicians who were responsive and caring and so we both rushed to the emergency room to meet the child. After an hour passed, we began to get anxious. We were afraid to leave for fear that Jack and his mother had met some dire fate in their haste to reach the emergency room. I began to regret that I had told them to hurry over in case that demand had precipitated some further calamity. Another hour passed and then another. With each passing moment, it became increasingly obvious that Jack's mother was not on her way. Finally, after nearly four hours had passed, Jack and his mother walked into the emergency ward of the hospital with big smiles and excited looks on their faces. The cut catheter hung from Jack's chest, its length considerably shorter than when I had last seen it. When asked where they had been for so long, Jack's mother replied that she had taken the toddler Christmas shopping. That afternoon had been the only time she had to shop, she told us. Since Jack was no longer bleeding, she thought she could wait just a little bit before bringing him in. She had no idea of the consternation she had caused and really was not too concerned when she found out. I guess we all define emergencies in our own unique ways. The line was repaired without difficulty but that surgeon was not as readily available the next time I called him for an emergency.

The prize for the most creative way to damage a catheter has to be given to Larry. Larry is now fourteen but was only seven when I first met him. He is hyperactive and has mental retardation due to a chromosomal defect. He also had ALL. Larry required a great deal of attention because of his behavioral and intellectual deficiencies. Despite his disabilities he performed fairly well at school but could be quite a handful when he got upset. Larry's mother was one of the most organized and thorough mothers whom I have ever met. She kept immaculate care of the boy's catheter. It lasted the entire three years of therapy without any complications. This was not easy since Larry was often curious about the catheter and liked to play with it. Somehow his mother kept his hands off the plastic tube enough so that it never became infected. Once chemotherapy is completed, most children will have their catheters removed. Larry, however, was not completely done with his need for the catheter even after the chemotherapy was finished. Shortly before he finished treatment of the leukemia, he developed some lung problems that required extensive evaluations. His mother requested that the catheter be left in place to make his care easier. One night, about one year after completing his leukemia therapy, Larry sneaked into his parent's bed and fell asleep. This was not unusual for him and so his mother merely rolled over and fell back to sleep. A few hours later she felt something warm in the bed next to her. She assumed that Larry had had an accident. This was also not a totally uncommon event. She turned on the light and was shocked to find out that the warm fluid in her bed was blood and not urine. Larry had bitten through the catheter. Fortunately, despite the horror movie appearance of the bed sheets, Larry had managed to lose very little blood. Still, I suspect that his mother and father lost several years off their lives that night. Larry had obviously decided that he wanted that catheter removed and he was not going to wait for a surgeon to do it. The line was removed in the conventional way the next morning. Larry continues to do quite well without one.

One of the major side effects of chemotherapy which make it frightening to many patients is nausea. Virtually everyone with a family member who received chemotherapy could tell a horror story about the nausea or vomiting that their loved one experienced. Sometimes the sickness was remembered as being worse than the cancer itself. Through the years, as chemotherapy treatments have become more intensive, so have the toxic side effects. Many techniques have been tried to control nausea and vomiting. Nausea and vomiting can have devastating effects on a person's life-style. It is hard to work or concentrate on school subjects, play, or even watch TV while suffering through severe nausea and vomiting.

Joshua is a case in point of the potential devastating effect of this negative reaction to chemotherapy. Joshua was diagnosed at age twelve with a large tumor on the back of his left leg. The cancerous tumor extended from the crease of his buttocks down to the back of his knee. The tumor was a *rhabdomyosarcoma*. This is a rare cancer that arises from muscle cells. Although nearly 60% of children who have this type of cancer will be cured, Joshua had several bad findings that made his chances of being cured much less. Shortly after his malignancy was first identified, Joshua's mother and father were told that the boy's leg might have to be amputated because the tumor was so big. His parents were so upset that they sought a second opinion. A different group of doctors recommended that Joshua receive intensive chemotherapy and radiation therapy according to a plan developed by the Intergroup Rhabdomyosarcoma Study. This international group is composed of doctors who have special expertise in the treatment of malignant muscle-cell cancers in children and adolescents.

Joshua started his therapy in another state. After completing the first twelve weeks of treatment, which included radiation therapy to his leg, he returned to continue the treatments here. I met him for the first time shortly after he returned from California. Every four weeks for two years, Joshua was admitted to the hospital to receive five days of chemotherapy. Even before he was admitted to the hospital, Joshua would begin to feel sick to his stomach. At first he would feel fairly well until a needle was placed in the reservoir of the implanted catheter in his chest. Just as soon as the needle was set in place, he would be overcome by waves of nausea. As time went on, he would become sick to his stomach just by entering the building in which my office was located. Finally, just seeing the street sign that indicated he was approaching the medical office building was enough for him to reach for an emesis basin. Once Joshua entered the hospital, he never said another word to me or to the nurses. He would receive medication to help him with the chemotherapy-induced nausea and vomiting which would sedate him. For the next five days, Joshua would awaken only long enough to spit saliva. He rarely, if ever, truly got sick from the chemotherapy itself. The medications used to control that problem seemed to work well.

It was his anxiety over the chemotherapy that caused him to become nauseated. This reaction is known as *anticipatory vomiting*. Anticipatory vomiting can be a serious problem. It has been reported to occur in as many as one out of every four people who receive chemotherapy. Agents used to treat nausea and vomiting are rarely effective at controlling this problem once it develops. Fortunately, newer medicines for controlling or preventing chemotherapy-induced nausea and vomiting have been developed. Some children now do not get sick at all from the same agents that made Joshua so ill. Since they do not get sick from the medicines, they do not get as anxious about the chemotherapy. Anticipatory vomiting is less likely to develop if there is nothing bad to anticipate. Joshua is now many years from his experiences, but he still reports mild nausea whenever he drives by the hospital building.

These newer and much more effective agents used to control nausea and vomiting were released for use within the past few years and have revolutionized the delivery of chemotherapy. They have made it possible to move much of the treatment of cancer to the outpatient department. It still amazes me to see a child eating a pizza while receiving a chemotherapy agent that just a few years ago would have caused the child to vomit for hours. Although these agents are fairly expensive, they are worth every penny. On the other hand there are a few agents used to treat cancer that actually increase the appetite. Children who are being treated for ALL get Prednisone or Decadron during the first month and often many times later as well. These medicines increase their appetite significantly.

I distinctly remember Emma, the very first child I ever took care of with ALL. She was a very pretty three-year old with luminous brown eyes and expressive features. Early on she was frustrated and frightened by all of the procedures necessary to treat the leukemia. Whenever any medical personnel would enter her hospital room, she would raise both her arms and brush her hands rapidly against the sides of her head. It was her way of telling them to go away. I would laugh whenever Emma would "brush" me off and would repeat the action towards her. As she became more comfortable with me, we would both make Emma's trademark signal and then laugh. By the third week of her therapy, Emma was feeling much better and was showing signs of bone marrow recovery.

New healthy cells were beginning to grow in place of the leukemia cells that had caused her to be ill in the first place. Emma's parents told me that the child's appetite was almost out of control, and they could hardly afford their food bill. I did not understand what they meant until

53

the next time they returned to the clinic. They told me that after leaving the clinic a few days earlier, they had gone to McDonald's where Emma had eaten 6 cheeseburgers. When they left McDonald's, they had then gone to Kentucky Fried Chicken where Emma had eaten a three-piece chicken dinner with all the trimmings. They had then headed home where Emma's mother had made more fried chicken for her still hungry child. I have not experienced anyone since with an appetite quite as voracious as Emma's. Still, some of the stories of large meals eaten or even of the cravings some of these children have while on Prednisone or Decadron are quite humorous. One child demanded filet mignon at 5 a.m. Another would eat ketchup all the time. One could not get enough pickles and vanilla ice cream. It was like living with a pregnant woman.

I spend a great deal of time discussing nutrition issues with parents when I talk to them about their child with cancer. If their child will be receiving Prednisone, they need to know what to expect or they may become frightened when they watch their child eat everything in sight. Sometimes the children will lose their appetites as one of the side effects of other chemotherapy agents. There are many supplements available that can be used to try to improve the appetite and prevent weight loss for these children. The healthier a child is during the chemotherapy, the better the quality of life.

Hair Machine

If one were asked to describe a patient with cancer, the most likely picture would include a head covered with wispy, nearly absent hair. No other characteristic associated with cancer and its treatment is as stereotyped or as common as this one. Hair loss is probably the least important side effect of treatment from a medical standpoint, but none can deny its emotional and psychological impact.

Radiation to the scalp will almost always result in significant hair loss but only in those areas that are within the radiation field. Many, but not all, of the chemotherapy medications result in hair loss, but the hair almost always grows back once the chemotherapy drugs are stopped. Sometimes the hair grows back even while further chemotherapy is being given. Return of the hair usually happens slowly. The hair that returns is often softer, curlier and, sometimes, even a different color than the hair which was lost. This change in hairstyle can sometimes be a source of anxiety. It was for George.

George was an 11-year old with straight, dark brown hair. He presented to his doctor with nosebleeds, which at first were fairly infrequent but then began to occur once or even twice each day. Because he also had a deep cough, his family doctor ordered a chest X-ray. The physician was quite surprised to find a large tumor sitting in George's chest just behind his breastbone. Within two days of the discovery of the chest tumor, George was in surgery. Fortunately, the surgeon had little trouble removing the large tumor. The tumor tissue was examined under a microscope and shown to be a malignant *germ cell tumor*.

A germ cell tumor is a cancer that arises from cells that were supposed to become sperm cells in boys and ova in girls. These cells become trapped in the baby's chest during development and never make it to the testicle or to the ovary. After the child is born, the trapped cells sometimes become cancerous. While treatment with radiation therapy is sometimes used for this type of cancer, I had concerns about using radiation with George. George's tumor sat just above his heart and lungs. Radiation given to the chest area can damage the heart and lungs. Since George was so young with his whole life in front of him, I chose to treat him with chemotherapy to try to avoid causing heart and lung difficulties later in life. George, like Joshua, developed a lot of anxiety and then anticipatory vomiting with the chemotherapy. After just four treatments, however, the tumor disappeared and therapy was stopped. The medicines used had caused George's hair to fall out shortly after he finished the first course of treatment. Within a few months of finishing the chemotherapy, George's hair began to grow again. Although he continued to have dark brown, almost black hair, his head was now covered with tight curls. When he came back for an examination three months following completion of the chemotherapy, the first thing he mentioned was how much he hated his curly hair. My comments about how cute his hair looked and how most women would pay large sums of money for permanents to make their hair look like his did not help. Marian then entered the room. She took one quick look at George's hair. She then walked over and ran her fingers through it.

"I love the feel of these curls," she cooed. "Do all the girls love it as much as I do?" Marian had touched his magic button. Looking cute with curly hair and girls were definitely the magic combination. He went away with a big smile on his face. Two years later the curls began to loosen and his hair again became straight. This distressed him as much as losing his straight hair had two years earlier. Somehow Marian convinced him that straight hair was what girls really liked. It has been seven years since George finished therapy. I am not sure what hairstyle he now has, but I am sure he is wearing his hair in whatever style he thinks will make him look handsome to the fairer sex.

The effect of hair loss on most younger children is minimal. They may comment on it or think that it is funny. One boy really liked the look. He said it made him look like Charlie Brown. He would call himself Charlie whenever he came in for chemotherapy. Some children tolerate hair loss even better than their parents do. Jami, for example, was a beautiful 3-year old with big brown eyes and rich, chocolate-colored hair that cascaded down to the middle of her back. Even at that tender age she took special care of her hair. Jami's hair fell out soon after she began chemotherapy to treat a *Wilm's Tumor*, a malignant tumor of the kidney. Her parents and I thought she would be traumatized. We certainly were. Jami's hair fell out virtually over night. One day she had a full head of hair and the next day all that were left were wisps. Jami was surprisingly unfazed. She laughed at her hair loss and said that she now looked like me. It was even better for her at home. Her older brother had often pulled her hair when she did something he did not like (which was usually all the time).

Shortly after returning from her initial hospitalization, Jami did something to make her older brother angry. He cried, "Don't do that again, Jami or I'll pull your hair!"

Her answer was, "Nyah, nyah, I don't have any so you can't pull it and so I can do whatever I want."

Although Jami was almost gleeful about her hair loss, some children are ambivalent. They may want to hide it from the world but do not seem terribly upset when it is finally exposed. Fred was 10 years old when his hair fell out shortly after he was started on radiation and chemotherapy to treat a *retinoblastoma*. A retinoblastoma is a malignant cancer that arises in the back of one or both eyes. Fred's retinoblastoma involved his right eye. Although Fred dealt with the hair loss fairly well, his parents still bought him a full scalp wig so he would not be embarrassed when in crowds or at church. Fred is one of the few boys for whom I have cared who has ever worn a wig. Most boys wear baseball caps or nothing at all on their heads. Fred would wear his wig every now and then but was very casual about it.

One day, while I was in my office seeing patients, Fred came in with his father. He sat down in a chair in the reception area. At just about the same time, my mother-in-law came to my office to visit me. She sat down next to Fred. In her usual friendly manner, she turned to the boy and started a conversation. The two chatted pleasantly for several minutes. My mother-in-law thought that Fred must be the brother of one of my patients since he had such a nice head of hair. She continued to believe that until about ten minutes later when Fred suddenly said, "Gosh, it's hot in here!" He then lifted the wig off his head and used it to fan himself. After a few seconds he replaced the wig acting as if nothing had happened.

My mother-in-law was not so sanguine. She had been a survivor of the Nazi concentration camps. The sight of bald children was very disturbing to her since it caused her to have flashbacks. She quickly excused herself and walked out of the room to regain her composure. If I did not love my mother-in-law as deeply as I did, I might have thought that the episode was funny. Instead, I very gently suggested to Fred that he be a little more careful as to where and when he removed his wig.

Some parents have shown amazing ingenuity when dealing with hair loss. One mother took advantage of her 3-year old daughter's smooth scalp on Halloween. She dressed her child as a moon maiden. The child's bald pate was the perfect touch. The child won a best costume award at a Halloween party and the mother was $50.00 richer as a result. Another child had her family paint a design on her scalp for Easter. She ended up resembling an Easter egg. I keep a picture of that child on a bulletin board of children's pictures I have collected over the years. Her picture is one I point to often since it shows that loss of hair does not have to be accompanied by a loss of a sense of humor. Sometimes, though, the hair loss raises the curiosity of strangers. This seems to be especially true of certain adults who have difficulty realizing that children can and do get cancer.

The same mother who used her child's hair loss to create a prize-winning costume told me this story. One day she and her little girl were shopping when an older gentleman walked up to her and asked why she had shaved her little boy's head. The fact that the "little boy" had earrings and a cute dress did not faze the rude observer.

"She has cancer. What's your excuse?" was all that the shocked mother could think to say. She knew she was being rude, but she figured that such a statement would get the man to recognize his error and apologize. Sorry to say, even that obvious reply did not deter the insensitive man. He continued to stare at the little girl. Finally, his embarrassed wife managed to move him away from the area before he made a further fool out of himself.

Teenagers seem to have the worst time dealing with hair loss. Teenagers have brittle egos anyway and much of their identity seems to be wrapped up in how they wear their hair. To be different is extremely difficult to most teenagers. It seems that their major goal is just to be one of the crowd. Cancer makes the teenager different. The further indignity of hair loss only adds insult to injury. For some teenagers, hair loss is even more difficult to tolerate than the cancer or the treatment. The world of a teenager today is not the world in which I grew up. It seems to be much harder and crueler. Baseball caps have become much more commonplace even among teenagers who are not hair-challenged. However, at some schools the color of the cap or just wearing a cap may be a gang symbol so caps have been outlawed. When a teenager who attends that school loses hair and returns wearing a baseball cap, the cap becomes a symbol of defiance even though that teenager has no desire to do anything to draw attention. Under such conditions, the teenager's desire to fit in ends up marking oneself as different.

Some of the cancer patient's fellow students may think they are being funny by pointing out the hair loss to other classmates or by tormenting the teenager with cancer about wearing a baseball cap in the classroom when no one else is allowed to do so. Even teachers sometimes contribute to the problem by calling attention to the teenager or to the cap. Most teenagers prefer not to have their hair loss pointed out. In that way, they can maintain their anonymity, normality and dignity. I try to teach the young men and women that hair loss is only external and that they still remain whole on the inside.

They usually respond, "How would you know?"

Since I have been bald since a fairly young age, I think I have a pretty good handle on dealing with hair loss. I try to get the teenagers to use humor to cope. I remember one young man who was disturbed about his looks after he lost his hair early during the treatment of ALL. I joked that he must have joined a gang since I knew of a few gangs that required their members to shave their heads. He was appalled that I would think that until he caught on to my teasing tone. He and I both knew that he was as far from being a skinhead as I was.

He looked at me and answered, "You must have joined the group, too." We both laughed. I truly enjoy it when someone can rise above their problems and see the humor in a difficult situation.

Gary represented a teenager who initially thought he would rather have cancer than lose his hair. He was 12 years old when I was called to see him. He had been admitted to the hospital with bad stomach pains. His doctor thought he had appendicitis. A surgeon was consulted and he was taken to surgery. When the surgeon opened the abdomen in the operating room, he encountered a large, widely-spread tumor. The tumor was a *lymphoma*, a cancer of the lymph nodes. A lymphoma—when it occurs in children—is a highly malignant and dangerous cancer, but children have a high cure rate. Once the diagnosis was confirmed, I spent several hours with Gary's mother and father explaining the disease and the treatment options. Gary was still too ill from the surgery and too groggy from pain medications to understand clearly what was happening. I explained to the anxious parents that their son would need to receive two years of chemotherapy. Gary's family had faced several difficulties over the previous year. The young man's father had a job with the civil service after he had spent more than 20 years in the Army. A heavy smoker, he had been diagnosed with lung cancer one year earlier. At that time, half of his right lung had been removed. Despite that, he continued to chain-smoke unfiltered cigarettes. Gary's younger brother was only 8 months old. At 4 weeks of life, he had been found to have a gaping hole between the right and left upper chambers of his heart. Because of that abnormal connection between the right and left sides of his heart, non-oxygenated blood flowed from the right atrium into the left atrium without first passing through his lungs as it was supposed to do. The blood with very low amounts of oxygen mixed with the normally oxygenated blood and decreased the amount of oxygen that the little boy could deliver to his tissues. The baby had a light blue color to his skin. He grew poorly and tired easily. Just sucking on his bottle would leave him weak, short of breath and sweating profusely. His pediatric cardiologist had planned on allowing him to grow big enough so that he could tolerate open-heart surgery. His mother had been taking him to his doctor in preparation for the heart surgery when Gary had developed severe abdominal pain. The discovery that Gary had a lymphoma and not appendicitis had put the surgical plans on hold. Despite all these events occurring in such a brief succession, both parents managed to retain an air of calm forbearance.

After a few days, Gary began to improve from the surgery. The pain medicines were decreased and I sat down at his bedside to discuss lymphomas and their treatment.

His first question to me was a simple. "Why me?" There is no good answer to this one. Some people would answer that the cancer is God's way of testing us, but that answer does not make good sense to me. What are we being tested for? Why would a just and righteous God need to test a religious, obedient, studious child who has never had a chance to explore the world? I answered in this way, "Gary, none of us have control over many of things that happen in our lives. Sometimes, no matter how good or honest or caring we are, unfair things do happen. When they do, we can waste time and energy trying to figure out why they happened or we can get our act together and make the situation as good as it possibly can be."

A diagnosis of cancer is a particularly difficult diagnosis to accept. Having cancer requires a person to look inside and realize that he or she is vulnerable and mortal. Bad things don't just happen to others; they have just happened to us. This concept is frightening and unnerving even for a mature adult. For a young man just facing his teenage years, a diagnosis of cancer can be overwhelming.

Gary was an exceptional young man with excellent values and strong self-confidence. He handled the information about the lymphoma very well. He asked appropriate and interesting questions that showed he understood the discussion. The conversation was peaceful and calm until I began to review the possible side effects of therapy.

"I won't lose my hair!" he yelled in anger and frustration. His statement was an expression of the importance of his hair to his self-image and not an indication of his determination to overcome that particular side effect. With that one vociferous comment, Gary turned his back on me as if to say that our discussion was concluded. He had said all he planned to say on that subject and any arguments further would be futile. All my attempts to get him to turn back toward me were unsuccessful. I left the room about 15 minutes later. I figured that I would give him a day to cope with the idea that he would have to temporarily lose his hair in order to beat the cancer. Things were only slightly better the next day. The anger was still there, but at least he listened while I talked. After reviewing much of the information we had covered the day before, I arranged a central venous catheter so that chemotherapy could start the very next day. He had no difficulty adjusting to the catheter and became actively involved in its care. However, he continued to be angry. He would barely speak to anyone while in the hospital, and this behavior continued even after he left to go home. By the time he started to come to the office for outpatient chemotherapy, his hair had already fallen out. His anger at what he considered to be an unfair and uncontrollable situation affected everyone around him. Finally, Marian sat him down. I think that her words were what got him to move beyond the anger to become an active participant in his treatment.

She said to Gary, "Dr. Lazarus and I did not cause your tumor. If we had that kind of power, you wouldn't have the cancer in the first place. We can't just wish this tumor away. It needs to be treated whether you like it or not. With the chemotherapy and prayer, we have a good chance to defeat this lymphoma. Still it's okay to be angry. I was angry when my sister got leukemia. But being angry at those who are here to help you or at the side effects of the medicines does not change the reality. You have a lymphoma. Be angry at the lymphoma and fight it with all your anger and strength."

Gary's attitude changed greatly shortly after that talk. That was fortunate since he still had a few hurdles to overcome. One of the chemotherapy medications that Gary was receiving was called *Vincristine*. Vincristine is made from the South American *vinca*, a very pretty flower. Vincristine is a very active chemotherapy agent, but one of its potential side effects is constipation. Sometimes, fortunately rarely, the constipation is so severe that the bowels actually stop for a short time. This was the side effect that Gary developed with the third dose of the drug. About three weeks after the chemotherapy was started, Gary's mother called in a panic. Gary was very sick with a high fever and severe headache. She had already called 911 and an ambulance was on the way to her house. She had just wanted me to know so that I could meet them there. By the time I arrived, he was having a seizure and his mother was working very hard to stay calm. Her face was white with fear as she watched her son writhe helplessly on the bed next to her. Gary was given medication to stop the seizures and then was transferred to the PICU as soon as he was stable. A CT scan of Gary's head was done as soon as he could safely be moved to the radiology department. A CT scan is a specialized X-ray that allows doctors to look inside various body structures without literally opening the body. The CT scan showed that Gary had an infection in the back part of his brain. A specialized study of Gary's heart using sound waves (an *echocardiogram*) was done. This showed a small ball of tissue hanging from the end of Gary's central venous catheter. Each heartbeat pushed the ball of tissue into the path of the blood flow as it journeyed through the heart. In addition, Gary had a small hole between the upper two chambers of his heart similar, but much smaller, than that which had produced problems for his younger brother. This hole had not been seen when his heart had been examined with an echocardiogram only a few weeks earlier. The source of Gary's problems was a series of unusual coincidences. He had developed a blood clot at the end of his central venous catheter. Bacteria had then started to grow in the blood clot. When Gary had developed severe constipation from the Vincristine, he had taken a big breath and tried to bear down to get his bowels to move. When he did that, a small piece of the infected clot had broken off. It then passed through the small hole in his heart into the arteries that provided blood to his brain. When the infection reached the back of his brain, it caused the brain cells to swell. The swelling was what had caused the teenager to have the seizure.

The first few days of treatment were critical. First, the central venous catheter had to be removed. That way, more pieces of the infected clot could no longer break off. Even before the catheter was out of his body, high doses of antibiotics were started. Gary was placed on strong anti-seizure medicines to prevent him from having any further seizures. The situation was made worse because Gary's brother had undergone open-heart surgery to correct his heart defect just one day earlier. He was in the PICU recovering from that surgery when Gary was wheeled in from the Emergency Room.

That evening, the infant lay in one bed with a multitude of tubes attached to various sites on his body while his ill older brother lay unresponsive in the very next one. The boys' weary mother sat in a chair between the two and tried her best to bring them a feeling of comfort that she sorely lacked. Fortunately, both young men did well and within a few days, both were on their way out of the PICU. Gary never had another catheter placed. Every two weeks for two years, he would receive chemotherapy through an IV placed each time in his arm. His brain healed completely as did his heart. Going through this experience made Gary aware of the realities of his disease and its treatment. He never again complained about his hair loss. At one point he told me that he thought that his cancer experience had made him a much more humble person. Gary is now a top student at an outstanding college. After some hard work we were able to convince the Marine Corps that Gary was not only cured of the lymphoma, but that he was also free of any other debilitating problems. At the end of his freshman year of college, Gary sent a letter to Marian and me thanking us for all that we had done to encourage and help him. I feel that Marian and I are the lucky ones since we were given the opportunity to get to know this fine young man. Hair loss was the major problem for Gary until he had to face truly significant complications that threatened his life.

Hair loss can happen suddenly or gradually within a few days or a few weeks. No matter how it occurs, it is always a reminder of the disease and its treatment. Someone once said, "When life deals you a lemon, make lemonade." There is no doubt that hair loss is a great big, crummy lemon. We do the very best we can to turn that lemon into large pitchers of lemonade.

Carla is a good example of someone who turned her hair loss lemon into a positive. Carla was 14 years old when I was first called to see her. She had endured headaches for a few months, which were getting progressively worse. When she began to vomit and walk unsteadily, her parents took her to a pediatrician in their hometown. That doctor found evidence for increased brain pressure and ordered a CT scan of the teenager's brain. Her doctor was not completely surprised when that study showed a large tumor arising in the back of her brain. It took nearly 9 hours before the neurosurgeon could completely remove the tumor. It took the pathologist a further three days of examination before he could be certain of the type of tumor that had been growing inside Carla's brain.

Carla's tumor was a highly malignant brain cancer known as an *ependymoma*. The quality and completeness of the surgery is the most important treatment for such a tumor. Radiation therapy seems to increase the chances that this kind of brain cancer will be cured. Whether chemotherapy adds anything to surgery and radiation therapy in increasing a child's chances of a cure is as yet unclear. I explained these facts as well as the possible side effects of radiation and chemotherapy to Carla's parents. After an extended discussion, we decided to treat the teenager with a combination of chemotherapy and radiation. Carla's parents were nice but very scared. They were convinced that their daughter was going to die. I told them that Carla could indeed die, but there was also a good possibility that she would live. I preferred to consider the positive possibilities since I truly had little control over which outcome would occur. All I could do was to give her the best therapy that was currently available and pray that she would be one of those who did well.

Carla handled the chemotherapy and radiation therapy treatments well. She barely became ill at all. The only side effect that truly bothered and depressed her was losing her hair. At the time of her diagnosis Carla had been attending a private school. Because she missed so much school during the first few months of her therapy, a school-provided teacher taught Carla at home. Carla liked home schooling. She could keep up with her schoolwork without having to face her classmates. She was frightened that they would tease her because of her hair loss. No teenager is ever brimming with self-confidence and Carla was no exception. She was not very secure about her looks or about her abilities. Her hair loss made her even more self-conscious. She had no desire to return to school even once she had reached a point in her treatment when it was not only feasible but desirable for her to do so.

The American Cancer Society has a wonderful program called, "Look Good - Feel Better." The program is run by local cosmeticians. These beauticians voluntarily supply their knowledge and their labor to make cancer patients look and feel better by teaching them how to wear wigs, scarves and make-up. In this way, the cosmeticians help the person maintain a sense of dignity while undergoing a treatment which is often dehumanizing and debilitating. Marian and I felt that Carla would greatly benefit from such a program, but we needed to convince her parents that it was all right for their daughter to wear a wig and make-up. Carla's parents were very strict. At age 14, Carla had never worn make-up. Carla's mother not only did not allow Carla to put on lipstick and eyeshadow, but she rarely wore any herself. It took a lot of convincing before her mother would allow the teenager to try on a wig and some very basic make-up. Finally, her mother agreed and the American Cancer Society was called. A date was selected when Carla would be in the office most of the day receiving chemotherapy. On the appointed day around the noon hour, a cosmetologist entered our office. I greeted her with profuse thanks and directed her to the bedroom in which Carla was resting while she received the chemotherapy. The door to the room was shut behind the cosmetologist. No one other than Marian was allowed into the room and she was only let in for brief periods to check the IV. Carla's parents, Marian and I waited anxiously outside in the hall for the cosmetologist to finish. Finally, we were all allowed into the room.

The results were stunning. The volunteer cosmetologist had found a wig with hair that closely matched Carla's original shade and texture. The style was short and stylish. It was secured in place with a hair ribbon that matched the color of her clothing. There was a touch of blush on her cheeks and she had a bit of color over her eyes as well as a pale lipstick. She looked beautiful. In just about one hour, she had transformed from a pale, sickly and sad teenager into a healthy, strong young woman. Carla could not have been more pleased. She could hardly stop beaming at herself in the mirror. A few days later she returned to school with renewed confidence. The next time she came back to the office, even her mother was wearing some make-up. Mother and daughter both seemed to have a new air of self-worth. Truly this was a triumph for both mother and daughter. Even now, 5 years later, Carla wears the wig and impeccable make-up. Last year, she graduated as an honor student from high school and has now entered college.

One of my favorite memories dealing with hair loss revolves around Paula. I met her a little over 9 years ago when she was diagnosed with *Hodgkin's Disease*. Hodgkin's Disease is a specific kind of lymphoma that arises in the lymph nodes. One of the peak ages for this cancer is the teenage years. As early as the mid-1960's, this cancer proved to be curable in a large number of patients. The ability to cure Hodgkin's Disease depends on how many lymph nodes are involved at the time of diagnosis, whether other organs other than lymph nodes are involved, how big the lymph nodes in the middle of the chest are swollen, and whether or not the person has systemic symptoms. Paula was found to have a very large lymph node riddled with the lymphoma on the left side of her neck. Further diagnostic studies showed the Hodgkin's Disease in lymph nodes in her chest as well as in her spleen.

When I first met Paula, she was 19 years old. She was a bright and energetic teenager with enormous enthusiasm and energy. She had not been feeling well for about two months before the swelling on the left side of her neck appeared. Her parents, who were very loving and protective, insisted that Paula see a doctor. It did not take long for the doctor who examined her to arrange a biopsy of the very large and firm node.

Paula's father was and is a very important lawyer in a nearby city. He approached his daughter's disease in much the same way he would have had she been an important case which he had to win. He studied the facts and reviewed the therapy options. He was very well-informed by the time that we sat down to make treatment decisions. After a grueling three hours of questions, answers and discussions, it was decided that Paula would receive a combination of chemotherapy and radiation therapy. I do not take care of many 19-year olds since most prefer to be cared for by doctors who specialize in treating adults with cancer. There are times when this is appropriate, but there are some cancers that occur in 19-year olds which are better handled by pediatric oncologists. Paula, however, did not have any difficulties with my pediatric background. She was charming, bright and sweet and she found me to be supportive, informative, helpful and caring. One of Paula's major concerns with the treatment was that it not interfere with her college education. I recommended that she take a lighter schedule during the 6 to 8 months she would be receiving therapy since I expected that the chemotherapy would make her tired. Still, I felt that staying in school with her friends would be excellent therapy.

Her other major desire was for everything to be done so she could retain her hair. It was easy to understand why Paula would not want to lose her hair. She had beautiful thick, blond hair that framed her face and accented her delicate features. Paula was very popular on campus, but she planned to tell only a few of her closest friends about her cancer. She was afraid that those who were not in on the secret might not understand if her hair suddenly fell out. We resolved to look for some technique that might allow her to keep her hair.

It is thought that decreasing blood flow to the scalp might help to decrease or even to prevent hair loss. The lower the amount of blood flowing through the scalp, the less the concentration of chemotherapy which reaches the hair follicles. This technique cannot be used in children with leukemia or with brain tumors because it might also decrease the amount of chemotherapy that gets to the cancer cells.

Two basic techniques have been tried to decrease blood flow to the scalp. One is to place a mechanical constriction around the head just below the hairline. I remember one child who had placed a tight rubber band around her head whenever she received chemotherapy. She claimed that her hair loss had been reduced by that elastic constriction of blood flow. I do not know whether that simple technique had actually helped that child, but I do know that she complained of headaches during each course of therapy. The second technique that has been tried to save cancer patients from hair loss is to cool the scalp. This was the technique Paula and I decided to try.

The first time she received chemotherapy, we placed ice bags around her head as she lay in bed. The technique was awkward and did not work well. The ice bags leaked and got her bed and clothes wet and cold but did not cool her scalp appreciably. After that first attempt at scalp cooling, I checked around for alternatives. The local hospital was testing a mechanical scalp cooler. I asked if I could borrow the instrument. The instrument involved more tubes and more preparation than almost anything else associated with Paula's treatment did, but she was willing to undergo the discomfort. The first time we used it, neither the hospital nurse nor I knew how it worked. The initial set-up was a bit of a comedy of errors, but, eventually, Paula had a cap on her head that became colder and colder as her chemotherapy was given. The machine consisted of a large tank of water and a freezing unit contained in a silver metal contraption about three feet long and two feet wide. The whole unit was on wheels as it was too heavy to lift. I never figured an easy way to fill up the water tank so I kept a small bucket in the office and filled up the water tank one bucket at a time. There were two hoses that left the contraption and connected to the back of a blue plastic shower cap. It was not really a shower cap. It was thicker and heavier than a normal shower cap. This was because the water from the tank was directed through the cooling unit where the temperature was lowered to near freezing. The water was then pumped through one hose into the shower cap. There it flowed through tiny tubes that ran through the cap and then exited through the second hose. The water then flowed back to the freezer unit to begin the cycle again.

In order to put this contraption on, Paula's hair had to be wet. We developed our own little routine. First, Paula put on a bathrobe with a towel around her neck. She would then bend over the sink in the bathroom and I would pour a plastic cup filled with lukewarm water on her hair. Once her hair was good and wet, Paula would pat it down to get rid of the excess water. She would then sit down in a recliner chair. A piece of cloth was placed over the wet hair, which was then covered by the shower cap. Following that, the hoses were then connected. Finally, with all that out of the way, we could worry about getting the chemotherapy ready.

After the ordeal we went through just to cool her head, running the chemotherapy was easy. Paula never complained that her head was too cold or that the cap was too heavy. She did, however, sit and shiver the whole time the cap was in place and running. I cannot truthfully say that the scalp icer really worked. Paula's hair thinned, but it never completely fell out. She always had enough hair that she could keep it nicely-styled. Few of her friends and none of her professors ever knew that she had Hodgkin's Disease and was receiving chemotherapy.

Would she have lost her hair if the cooling device had not been used? I really do not know. I have not used the device since and do not believe that the hospital kept it. Still, a hair-saving device or medicine that truly worked would be terrific.

Faith

Faith is the belief in something outside ourselves that gives us strength at times when events around us seem hopeless. Faith plays an important role in helping people cope with serious illnesses. Studies have shown that women with breast cancer who have positive attitudes have better outcomes than women with breast cancer who are pessimistic about their chances.

Faith in the doctor who is providing the treatments and in the treatment itself is extremely important. For some disorders, just the belief that the treatment will work is enough to result in significant improvement in the underlying condition. This effect of faith is known as the *placebo effect*. The placebo effect tells us that, for some diseases and for some people, a belief that a cure will work is as effective as any medicine. Even if the placebo effect does not have any impact on the condition itself, it might help improve the patient's spirits and quality of life. Patients who feel better take care of themselves better.

It is known that a patient who has better nutrition while undergoing cancer therapy tolerates the treatments easier and with fewer side effects. Faith can therefore help patients make it through radiation and chemotherapy without as many difficulties. Faith alone is not enough, but the lack of faith in anything can prove to be destructive. Unfortunately, there is no way to measure or to charge for faith and so it has little importance to the financiers and economists who currently are running modern medical care. One of the more damaging effects of managed care is to force patients to switch doctors frequently or to make access to specialists more difficult. This undermines the person's faith that their care is the best that it can be and decreases the impact of faith.

Some children with cancer will be cured. Others with the same type of cancer will initially respond, but then the cancer will return and the child will die. Despite all the systems designed to predict who will live and who will die, there really is no way to know. Some people suggest that faith in God plays a strong role. I do believe that there is an outside force much more powerful than myself, which is important in the care of children with cancer. A belief in God is very healthy and helpful to parents struggling with the diagnosis of cancer in their child. Faith gives strength and comfort. It gives some sense of control when the cancer diagnosis has set one's world spinning out of orbit. It provides an inner core of serenity when everything else is in chaos. A belief in a being far more powerful and knowledgeable than any person could possibly be provides a sense of peace, but I do not believe that prayer by itself can change the course of a child's disease. I find that idea to be arrogant and inconsistent with a rational view of the world.

When my sister-in-law was struggling with leukemia, my family and I prayed very hard that she would be relieved and cured of her disease. Despite our fervent desires, the leukemia eventually killed her. When another family announced that their loved one was healed because of their prayers, all I could feel was anger. What made their prayers better than ours? Why would God answer one person's prayers and not another's? It became clear to me that such a belief was arrogant. It presumed that people have different importance in the eyes of the Lord. I cannot accept that.

The God in whom I believe treats all human beings as equally important. God does not specifically answer individual prayers for healing. To do so would be to interfere with the natural order of life and create chaos. In addition, it would create two classes of people—those who have God's ear and those whose prayers are ignored.

Ashley helped me understand how religion could both help and also hurt. Ashley had been fine until a few days before I first met her when she began to vomit and complain of headaches. She was seen by her pediatrician who noticed that she was walking unsteadily and arranged for her to have an MRI of the brain. The MRI showed a large tumor arising from the left side of the little girl's brain. Within 24 hours she was on the operating table and the tumor was being removed. Because of its size and location, the tumor could only be partially removed. Following the surgery I was contacted and asked to see her. I walked into the PICU and had no problem recognizing her. She was sitting up in one of the hospital beds. White gauze bandages were wrapped around her head so that it looked like she was wearing a turban. Not a wisp of hair could be seen. The child had light blue eyes that were wide and bright. From that first day and every time I saw her after that, she always seemed to have a big smile on her face. She recovered quickly and was soon moved to a room on the pediatric floor. Within a week of the surgery she was ready to start chemotherapy and radiation therapy. After the first course of chemotherapy in the hospital, she was able to go home. She received the next several treatments as an outpatient.

About six months into therapy, a repeat MRI study showed that the tumor had shrunk significantly in size. Except for a rim of remaining tissue, the tumor had been completely eliminated. I was very happy with the results and I took the mother into my office to discuss the MRI scan with her. Most parents are usually ecstatic when they hear such news. Ashley's mother was nonchalant. When I asked why she did not seem excited or encouraged by the MRI scan, she responded that the past weekend she had taken her daughter to a religious revival. The minister had laid his hands on the child and announced that he had cast out the devil that had been responsible for the brain tumor. Ashley' mother was secure in her belief that the tumor was cured and she did not need an MRI scan to prove to her what she felt deeply. The woman was so sure that her daughter had been cured by the faith healer that she refused any further chemotherapy. I did not agree with stopping the therapy, but I had little choice. I only asked her if I could continue to see the child and monitor her progress.

I continued to see Ashley at regular intervals. When she would come in for a visit, her mother would talk with other parents. She would tell them with great conviction how the faith healer had cured her child and tried to convince them that they should take their children to the same minister. Her passion for her belief was disconcerting to many of the parents. They would complain privately to Marian or me that Ashley's mother was making them uncomfortable. Soon I had to have Ashley come to the office when no other families were present to avoid confrontations. About two years after I first met and began treating Ashley, an MRI scan showed definite evidence that the tumor was growing again at the original site. Ashley's mother reacted with appropriate sadness and disbelief. I truly did not know how she could reconcile her belief in her child's physical cure by the faith healer with the reality seen in black on white on the MRI scan. Did the return of the tumor mean that the faith healer had failed or that the mother had failed by somehow not maintaining her faith? I feel that the faith healer placed himself into a no-lose situation. If the tumor never grew back, it was because of the success of the faith healer. If the tumor did grow back, he could always claim that he had cured the child, but the mother's or child's lack of faith had allowed the tumor to grow back. In Ashley's case, her mother's faith allowed her to cope with the awful news that her daughter had a brain tumor. It gave her enormous strength and hope. That is the beauty and greatness of religious belief. The faith healer, however, gave her false hope. He encouraged her to abandon the standard therapy. While the standard therapy did not guarantee a cure, it at least gave provable odds to the mother and might have allowed her to deal realistically with her child's situation.

Christian was a 3-year old boy whom I became involved with during my days in the Air Force. He was the epitome of a healthy, active child until he began to complain that his legs hurt. His very attractive, attentive parents did not think the problem was too serious until the little boy began to limp. When he refused to stand on his right leg a few days later, they brought him to the Air Force clinic for evaluation. Studies showed that the thighbone was being eaten away by a malignant disease. The general pediatrician who had first examined the boy asked me to see the boy in consultation. Within a few days it became clear that the boy had tumors in many more sites than just his leg bone. He had a primary tumor in his abdomen known as a *neuroblastoma*.

The tumor had spread wildly throughout the child's bones and bone marrow. The treatment for neuroblastoma in those days was chemotherapy, but the results were dreadful. Many of the children would initially respond but within several months, the cancer would recur and the child would eventually die. A newer treatment involving bone marrow transplant was looking promising. I suggested to the parents that if Christian had a good response to initial therapy, I would arrange for him to have a bone marrow transplant performed at another center.

They agreed and therapy was started. Like many other children, Christian's neuroblastoma began to shrink from the effects of the chemotherapy. Within a few weeks of starting therapy, he was up running and playing as if he had never had anything wrong. After about six months of treatment, I could find no evidence of the disease in any of the boy's studies. I sent the child and his parents to another state where there was a treatment center that was pioneering the bone marrow transplant technique. A few days later the family reappeared in my office. I was surprised to see them back so soon.

Christian's parents explained that they had been scared by the possible side effects of the bone marrow transplant and they had declined for their son to participate. I had told them that neuroblastoma usually only gave us a very brief window of opportunity before it returned and Christian's tumor proved no different. Christian began complaining of leg pain and limping less than a week after the family returned from their trip. There were other, less effective treatments that I offered, but the parents declined all of them. I then offered them hospice care.

During our conversation about hospice care, they told me that they had joined a church that believed that true physical cures could be obtained if the family had enough faith. This admission bothered me. One of the facts of hospice is that all participants must deal with the reality that the child has a disease that is not going to be cured by conventional means and that most likely the child is going to die. If the parents believed that Christian would be physically healed of his disease, then the presence of the hospice nurses and myself trying to get them to cope with the reality that their child was probably going to die would be contrary to that belief. When their child died, their anger at his death might be turned against those who did not share their belief in the physical healing by faith. I was concerned that the hospice program and the hospice workers might get hurt in such a situation and I withdrew the offer of hospice. I told the family that I did not agree with their beliefs but I did not want to interfere in any way with their faith. I promised to help them and Christian. I explained that Christian would need to be admitted to the hospital if his condition worsened and he needed more support. In spite of the parent's deepest wishes and faith, Christian did not progress. Nearly every day the family home was filled with members of the church. They would pray over Christian nearly constantly. Whenever either of the parents would express any doubts, one of the congregants would take that parent aside and persuade them to return to their belief.

As time passed, the boy's pain worsened. I ordered morphine for him, but the members of the church would not let the parents give it to the child. Pain was a sign that the tumor was not going away. Since the parents had to have constant faith that God was physically healing their little boy, they had to believe that the pain was actually going away. The parents were torn between their deep faith and the obvious evidence that their child was suffering. Because of their ambivalence, members of the church took the child away from the parents for a week. He was given no pain relief for the entire week. His suffering must have been terrible. Finally, the parents could stand it no longer and asked that he be admitted to the hospital for intravenous medications. The scene in the hospital was difficult for the nurses and me. The hospital room was filled with church members at all times of the day and night. There was hardly any room in which to move or to breathe. Prayers were constantly being said around the boy's bed. Within a short time of Christian's admission, he became unresponsive. A few hours later, he stopped breathing and was at peace at last. I could barely get into the room to see the child or to comfort his parents.

The church minister took me aside and said, "We never had lost one before."

The arrogance of that statement astounded me. What an amazing church—they had defeated death itself. Christian's mother sat with her child in her lap like a living Pietá for a long time. She firmly held to the belief that her child would awaken and be healed, but it was not to be. Finally, he was taken from her and transported to the funeral home. I did not attend Christian's funeral. I was told by a few nurses who were there that the ritual was interesting and quite moving. The nurses said that the boy's body had not been handled well by the funeral home. His face retained a pasty white color. They could see the marks made where the embalming fluid had been applied. They were appalled at how poorly the funeral home had done its work. Christian's parents were also very angry at the funeral home. Later, however, they had a different view. Christian's mother still believed that he would awaken and come back to life even at the funeral service. It took the obvious signs left by the funeral home to convince her that her child had truly died and was not going to come back.

Despite my experience with Ashley and with Christian, I believe that religious support at the diagnosis and throughout the treatment of a child with a malignancy is quite valuable. The pastoral service at a hospital provides people who are willing to listen without judgment to families in crisis. I have had wonderful experiences throughout my career working with many wonderful rabbis, priests and ministers who have given of themselves to help these families.

One of the most important lessons that I have been able to obtain from my experiences with families and with clergymen and women is how important it is to listen to the concerns of the parents and the children. People often do not say what they mean and sometimes do not mean what they say. It is important to listen carefully to the words as well as to their meaning in order to provide the best care to each child. When a parent calls with a concern about a child, it requires great attention to detail and the ear of experience to distinguish minor problems from potentially dangerous ones. Sometimes it is the tone of voice used by the parent or the way in which they describe the events that make me feel that things may be worse than described. Some parents do not realize the gravity of a situation. On the other hand, some parents panic at every little change and this too must be recognized. It takes some time to get to know each family and what creates anxiety for them.

Each telephone call is important and must be listened to carefully. I truly believe that listening is one of the most important medical skills. Lindsay represents a good example where a major infection initially sounded like a minor problem. Lindsay was an almost 2-year old whose ALL had not responded as quickly as desired to the initial chemotherapy. As a result she had been placed on a much more intensive treatment. After 4 months of therapy, however, she was doing very well and in an excellent remission. Lindsay was a beautiful and bright child with a strong will and a stubborn streak. She loved for me to look in her ears during an examination because I would whistle like a bird or bark like a dog or meow like a cat and pretend that one of those animals had found its way into her ears. She thought that activity made her very special and I thought so too. Her mother was a single mother who had a very supportive family. Lindsay's mother had been well on her way to a degree as a licensed vocational nurse when her daughter was diagnosed with leukemia.

Five months after therapy started, Lindsay entered a new phase of therapy, which called for chemotherapy to be given by mouth, intravenously, and by shots in her legs. The medicine given by mouth was *Dexamethasone*.

Dexamethasone, especially when given three times daily for three weeks in fairly high doses, produces marked weight gain along with swelling of the face and the abdomen. The swelling of the face is called a moon face because the face ends up looking like a full moon. Towards the end of her three weeks of Dexamethasone, Lindsay looked like a large beach ball with a smaller but just as round ball on top. Her arms and legs looked tiny in comparison to her swollen body. She could only waddle when she walked and was short of breath whenever she lay down because her enlarged stomach would press up against her lungs. Despite these changes, she seemed happy and continued to play as before. On the last week of the Dexamethasone therapy, I saw Lindsay in my office. I saw no significant changes other than the marked weight gain. The one thing that I did notice was a tiny pink area on her stomach just above her diaper line. Her mother told me that the tape of the elastic disposable diaper had caught on the child's skin earlier that morning. She did not seem to be the least bit concerned and the area did not seem to bother Lindsay at all.

About two days later I called just to make sure that Lindsay was all right. Her mother told me that she had not noticed any big change in her child except that she seemed to be a bit more irritable and that the pink area on her lower abdomen now looked like a dark purple bruise. Dexamethasone is well known to produce irritability. I know that I would be irritable if I looked like a beach ball and had difficulty walking. But the words, "dark purple bruise" set off a red flag in my mind. If the bruise had occurred two days earlier when I first saw it, the dark purple color should be fading. Perhaps what her mother thought was a bruise was something else.

"Why don't you bring Lindsay in so that I can take a look at that bruise?" I asked trying to keep any hint of concern out of my voice so that Lindsay's mother would not panic. I was not certain that my suspicions were correct.

I was very glad that I had told Lindsay's mother to bring her daughter in for an examination. The area that had been a pale pink two days earlier was now a deep purple. Even though the spot was no bigger than a dime and Lindsay looked as contented as she usually did, I knew that the sore represented trouble. In very short order, Lindsay was admitted to the hospital and antibiotics were started. I called an infectious disease specialist since this bruise did not look like a bruise but neither did it look like a run-of-the-mill infection. Just as I feared, the spot slowly grew in size and the purple color deepened. Soon it was a quarter-sized purple-black sore. Shortly afterward a blister developed in its center. The antibiotics suggested by the infectious disease specialist did not seem to be touching the sore. After three days the lesion had grown big enough that I called a plastic surgeon to take a look.

The plastic surgeon suggested that the site looked like the little girl had been bitten by a brown recluse spider. This poisonous spider is found in the southern United States. It is recognized by a design on its back in the shape of a violin. The bite of the spider is fairly innocuous and at first the person may not be realize that he or she has been bitten. Slowly, during the next few days, the initial bite site slowly enlarges and the skin tissues in the area begin to die from the effects of the injected poison. That certainly fit the description of what was occurring on Lindsay's abdomen. Three days after the original phone call, Lindsay was taken to surgery. An area about four times the size of a fifty-cent piece was removed from over her abdomen. The skin down to the muscle had to be cleaned off because it was full of dead tissue.

The plastic surgeon still believed that the problem was due to a spider bite until the pathologist found that the dead tissues contained a very dangerous fungus known as *mucormycosis*. This fungus is highly invasive and nasty especially in people whose immune systems are not functioning properly. *Decadron* is a major suppressor of the immune system. Lindsay had somehow become infected with a fungus that was potentially lethal. Fortunately, by aggressively responding to the mother's phone call, we were able to control and eventually eradicate this dangerous infection. Lindsay has now been off all leukemic therapy for over two years. The only remaining sign of her ordeal is an abnormality the size of a half-dollar in the skin of her abdomen.

It is the ability to recognize such situations and react appropriately that marks an astute clinician. Still, despite years of training, extensive experience and a high degree of suspicion, even the finest physician will occasionally miss the often-subtle clues that differentiate a minor problem from a potentially fatal one.

Jennifer, too, was another child where cues given to me over the phone caused me to alter my plans of treatment. Jennifer was a pretty 5-year old who also had ALL. She had been in remission for one and a half years and was doing very well. At least two times each year, I go to a meeting out of town to meet with doctors and other specialists who deal with children with cancer. I left Marian behind to serve as an initial screener and had another oncologist available to deal with any problems that might arise with my patients. Jennifer's mother called Marian on my second day away and said that Jennifer had a high fever. Jennifer's mother rarely called about problems and so Marian knew that something had to be seriously wrong with the child for her mother to be so worried. Jennifer's mother wanted the child to be seen by me but I was not available. Marian suggested that the oncologist who was covering my practice could see Jennifer, but her mother did not know him and was uncomfortable with that idea. Marian then suggested that Jennifer be seen by the pediatrician who had first diagnosed the leukemia. Later that same day Jennifer's mother called Marian in a panic. Jennifer had been seen by that pediatrician earlier in the day and had been told that there was nothing wrong with her child. When the child continued to have a high fever and complain of malaise, the mother had called the pediatrician and been told that she was a nervous mother and to stop calling. She still did not want the covering oncologist to see her daughter.

Marian reached me at my hotel room that evening. She told me that she had not seen the girl, but she knew Jennifer's mother and knew that something was wrong. I was not due to return for two more days but the anxiety in Marian's voice convinced me that I needed to change my plans. I was able to arrange a flight out and arrived home the next day at noon. I went straight from the airport to my office where Jennifer and her mother were waiting. As soon as I saw her, I knew that I had made the right decision. According to the child's mother, she did not look any different than she had for the past two days but to me she appeared to be very ill. A chest X-ray done once she arrived at the hospital showed that Jennifer had pneumonia. Antibiotics were instituted and within 48 hours the child felt much better. The quick actions and instincts that led Marian to realize that Jennifer was truly ill undoubtedly saved the child's life. Jennifer will be entering high school this fall with no evidence that she ever had leukemia or pneumonia.

Listening is an important, but, unfortunately, rarely well learned or used skill. There are no classes in medical school on how or when to listen. Listening is the most important part of taking a history and understanding what a patient is actually feeling and trying to say. Unfortunately, managed care has decreased the amount of time that most doctors spend with their patients. Active listening is becoming a much rarer art these days. Sometimes patients do not even get to visit with a doctor but only with a physician's assistant or a nurse practitioner. The physician's assistant or nurse practitioner may be very good listeners. Many people, however, are not comfortable sharing intimate medical details with someone who has not gone to medical school. Even when a doctor listens carefully to what the patient is saying, the doctor may have already come to some conclusions about what is wrong with the patient based on incomplete facts. Many doctors have already made the diagnosis before they have even seen the patient. I must admit that there have been occasions when I also have been guilty of this same practice.

Some disorders present so classically that just a few brief details allow a complete diagnosis. Still, it is important to realize that each patient brings an individual twist to the same disease. I was once called by a pediatric cardiologist one evening after I had left my office for the day. He wanted to describe a patient to me about whom he was concerned. The child was 4 years old and had been having problems breathing whenever he lay down. A chest X-ray had been obtained on the child and had showed a large mass in the middle of the boy's chest.

He started to go on with his description but I stopped him and said, "That child has a lymphoma. Hold everything until I get there."

The cardiologist explained that there were five doctors there and they were ready to take the child to open-heart surgery. I repeated that he was to stop any plans for surgery and that I would be there right away. I hurried as fast as I could considering that I had to buck rush hour traffic. I walked into the room where the boy was being evaluated. The back of the boy's hospital bed was straight up. The child sat in the bed and had a look of anxiety on his face. His parents flanked him on either side. Standing around the bed were four doctors. One was the cardiologist who had called me. The other three doctors included a cardiac surgeon, an anesthesiologist and a pulmonary specialist. About 20 minutes earlier the pulmonary specialist had removed some fluid from the boy's chest cavity.

Almost as soon as I entered the room and introduced myself to the boy and his parents, the child's father asked me, "What is wrong with my child?"

I told him, just as I had the cardiologist, that I felt that his child had a lymphoma. Not more than a minute passed before one of the hospital pathologists stepped through the doorway. The pathologist announced to all present that based on what he was observing in the chest fluid that the child clearly had a lymphoma. The cardiologist turned his gaze from the pathologist toward me and gave me a look of admiration. He was astonished that I could make a diagnosis of a malignant lymph node cancer over the phone without ever seeing the patient or the X-rays. I did not tell him that his description of the child's condition was classic for that type of lymphoma because I wanted him to retain his awe at my amazing diagnostic powers. Fortunately, the child responded extremely well to chemotherapy and continues to be happy and healthy 9 years later.

There are few occasions when a patient presents with textbook symptoms and signs and can be diagnosed over the telephone. Many times, however, the facts that are presented by the patient do not match any preconceived notion of what might be wrong. One must have good listening skills to realize when the facts do not match the presumed diagnosis. This may require rethinking the original idea or realizing that each person often adds his or her own twists onto even classic signs and symptoms. Many times what the patient or the parent says is not as important as what is not said.

Parents who come to my office for a consultation are already scared when they walk through the front door. A pediatric oncologist is something like a dentist. He or she may be the nicest person in the whole world, but because a dentist deals with things that might be painful, visits are often dreaded. Many parents have told me while leaving the office after being told that their child does not have cancer that they liked me, but they hoped that they would never have to see me again. I do not take such statements personally since I would feel exactly the same way if I were in their shoes.

The parent who brings his or her child in because the child is pale or bruising easily is usually fearful that my diagnosis will be leukemia. The mother who asks me why her child might be having headaches is thinking that her child might have a brain tumor but is afraid to say the words out loud in case that might make her thoughts come true. I find that by addressing these fears directly at the start of a visit that a great deal of the anxiety can be diffused.

I remember once when Marc's mother called me at 2:00 am. Marc was a 4-year old boy who was being treated for ALL. He had been in remission for one full year when she called. Marc had suddenly developed a high fever. Fevers are not uncommon in children let alone children who are being treated for leukemia, but children on therapy for leukemia are more apt to have something serious and need to be seen quickly. As Marc's mother continued to describe the child's symptoms early that morning, I was remembering what his symptoms had been when he had first been diagnosed with leukemia. The description she gave was very similar. I asked her to bring the boy to my office right then. I do not usually have patients come to my office at such strange hours, but I felt that I could get an answer quicker than if they had gone to the Emergency Room. Marian rolled over and groaned as I hung up the receiver. I kissed her and told her I would be back as soon as I could. I dressed as quickly as I could in the dark so as not to disturb her.

I met Marc and his mother about one hour later. The office building was dark and somewhat foreboding at that early hour of the morning. Marc looked sick. I drew his blood and got the blood counting machines started as quickly as I could. I felt my heart sink as I watched the number of white cells rise well above normal. It took about fifteen minutes before a smear of his blood had gone through the stainer. The elevation in the white blood cell count could be due to infection, but I was afraid that the cells I would see would be leukemic. With a slight tremor to my hands, I picked up the stained slide. I put it under the lens and focused the microscope. With a deep sigh of relief I realized that the elevated cell count was due to Marcel's normal response to an infection. The slide was filled with normal white cells with not a single leukemic cell present. I walked back to the treatment room where Marc and his mother sat waiting.

With a big smile on my face, I announced, "All I see are normal cells. Marc is not having a leukemia relapse."

Marc's mother surprisingly replied, "Well, why would you be worried about that?"

I guess it is sometimes possible to guess wrong about what is bothering a parent. Despite Marc's mother's lack of concern, I try to put myself in the position of the parents. This helps me to share their fears. When a child complains of symptoms that remind the parents or myself of the original symptoms, I feel that tests need to be done as soon as possible to prove that the original cancer has not recurred. Sometimes the brothers or sisters of the child with cancer develop symptoms that remind their parents of the symptoms that originally led to the cancer diagnosis.

The anxiety that another child in the family might have cancer can be overwhelming. It may affect everything the parents do until they are reassured that the symptoms are not due to cancer. Siblings of children with cancer are at a slightly increased risk to develop some sort of cancer themselves. Because of this increased risk, I do recommend screening tests for the siblings if the parent's anxiety has become too great. It is unusual for a pediatric oncologist to have to take care of more than one family member with some sort of cancer. It is known, however, that in some families there is an inherited risk to develop cancer. Children whose mothers or fathers or other family members appear to have inherited one of these cancer genes need to be watched closely. In that way if a cancer does develop, it can be found early when it is most likely to be curable.

Larry, the boy who bit through his catheter, was the son of a man who had been diagnosed with a cancer of the lymph nodes four years earlier. Gary's father had been diagnosed with lung cancer one year before his son was discovered to have a lymphoma, but the father was a heavy smoker and the two cancers may not have been associated. However, there are some studies that suggest that people who are exposed to second-hand tobacco smoke may be at a higher risk to develop certain malignancies. Billy's father had been diagnosed and successfully treated for a cancer of his testicles a few years before Billy was treated and cured of leukemia.

Are such cases linked by heredity? Scientists are beginning to find some answers to explain who may be at risk to develop cancer. Tests are not yet readily available that can distinguish those who are at risk from those who are not. Even when they do become available, many questions will be raised. How should someone who carries the abnormal gene be screened? What will be the best age at which someone should be screened? Who will have access to the information? Will people truly want to know that they carry a cancer gene when treatment for the disease is still not good? Will people who carry cancer genes be able to get jobs or insurance once their risk is made known to prospective employers or insurance carriers? The questions and dilemmas raised by these cancer genes seem almost insurmountable. It will be more important to find some means to decrease the risk or to treat the cancer more effectively than just to know that someone is at risk. We are a long way off from being able to accomplish those feats.

One of the more dramatic examples of multiple cancers occurring in more than one member of the same family happened while I was serving in the Air Force. Leonard came to the Air Force clinic with complaints of headache, vomiting and weakness on his left side. The Air Force pediatrician who examined him quickly recognized that Leonard had a serious problem. He arranged for the boy to have a CT scan of his brain that same afternoon. If Leonard were to present today, an MRI scan would be the best test, but MRI's were not available at that time. The CT scan showed that Leonard had a *brain stem glioma*.

The brain stem is a portion of the brain that is critical to the basic functioning of the body. Right in the center of the brain stem is the *pons*. Leonard's pons was swollen and very abnormal in appearance. A brain stem glioma is a devastating tumor. Because of the vital structures found in the brain stem, a tumor in the pons has disastrous consequences on neurological functioning. Surgery for these tumors is almost never indicated because there is no way to remove the tumor without destroying vital parts of the brain. Radiation therapy has had limited success. It can increase the duration of survival, but in most cases radiation does not increase the chance of cure. Chemotherapy has not yet been demonstrated to play much of a role in the care of children with brain stem gliomas. Pediatric oncologists and neurosurgeons probably fear this tumor more than any other because there are such poor treatment options. Most children with a brain stem glioma will die within one year of diagnosis.

Leonard was sent first to an Air Force neurosurgeon and he sent the boy to see me. Leonard was the youngest of four children. He had one full brother who was two years older. The oldest children, a half-brother and a half-sister, shared the same father with the two younger boys. Leonard was a handsome 8-year old with an air of courage and determination. He looked like a child one would see in a commercial for some major product. He had an appealing, warm look that made him instantly sympathetic and believable. He had blond hair and crystal blue eyes. Even after the diagnosis of this terrible disease, he retained an air of peace that calmed those who came into his presence. It was this almost supernatural serenity that allowed those around him to continue to hope that the tumor would be controlled even when we were all fairly certain what the eventual outcome would be.

Six months after I became involved in his care and five months after completing radiation therapy, the tumor began to grow again. Leonard's mother had used the six months to deal with the reality of her child's condition and she refused any further therapy. Leonard's symptoms, which had improved following the radiation therapy, returned with a vengeance. His left leg became weaker until he lost the ability to walk.

The left side of his mouth lost its tone and drooped at the corner. He drooled frequently and uncontrollably. His speech slowly and steadily deteriorated until he became only barely intelligible.

After the recurrence of the tumor was diagnosed, Leonard had asked for a trip to Disneyworld. This was arranged through the generosity of the Make-A-Wish Foundation. The trip was a tonic for the family. Even though Leonard spent most of the trip in the hotel pool, he still had a wonderful time. I visited the family home a few days after they returned. While there I asked the children to draw me some pictures of their trip. Each of them grabbed some paper and crayons and went happily to work while I talked with Leonard's mother and father. Leonard's picture was full of scribbles since he was unable to hold his crayons steady. His siblings all drew pictures that showed a happy family enjoying the sights of central Florida. Those pictures were important to me because they told me how special and meaningful that trip had been for Leonard's family.

Over the next few weeks I visited the home about three or four times to check on the young man and to support his family. His mother was terrific. She was scared and unsure what to do for her dying child, but she managed to provide him with what he needed most; love and security. Leonard died without pain and without a struggle at home. I was not ashamed to cry freely as I gazed upon the lifeless body of a child who to me epitomized the joy of living. I stayed in contact with the family for more than a year after Leonard's death but gradually we lost contact with each other. The family seemed to adjust to the loss of their son and brother as well as one could expect. A few years later I left the Air Force to establish a private practice. I had not heard from Leonard's family for a good while, but I thought of them from time to time. Leonard's picture occupied a central place on a bulletin board that I kept on a wall in my new office. The bulletin board was filled with pictures of some of the children I have cared for through the years. Every now and again I would look at Leonard's picture and remember what he, his family and I had gone through together.

One evening I received a page to call someone whose name I did not recognize. As soon as I heard the voice on the other end, I knew that it was Leonard's mother. Her last name had changed because she had divorced and remarried since I had last seen her. I was thrilled to hear from her. I asked how the children were doing and she filled me in on the happenings of her older two stepchildren. When I asked her about the now youngest boy, she hesitated. I asked her again thinking that I might have called him by the wrong name.

She answered in a quiet, barely discernible voice, "Jordan has just been diagnosed with a malignant brain tumor."

I was stunned. What was there to say under such circumstances? Only a few years after burying one child, this mother faced the prospect of watching another son die. Jordan was now 14 years old. He was a bright teenager with a marvelous sense of humor and was well aware of the severity of his illness. He was physically a more mature version of his younger brother. His mother had called me to see if I would take on Jordan's care. I readily agreed. There are few cancers in childhood that can rival Leonard's brain stem glioma for grimness of prognosis. As difficult as it was to believe, Jordan had one of them. His treatment consisted of surgery, radiation therapy and chemotherapy.

Through all of the difficult treatments, the young man retained his sense of humor and his deep religious faith. Just like Leonard's cancer that initially responded only to grow again later, Jordan's cancer initially shrank but within several months had recurred. Once again, his mother decided on no further therapy and a hospice was set up to allow the teenager to remain at home. This hospice was far more difficult and emotionally draining than hospice was for Leonard. This time we not only had to deal with Jordan, who was completely aware of the changes that were happening to him, but also with his family who had lived through all of this before.

I asked his mother later how she could ever find the strength to handle such immense and painful tragedies.

Her answer was simple. "I didn't know that I had a choice. If I had had a choice, I would have chosen a trip to Hawaii."

As would we all.

Acceptance

The people who go to medical school come from many different backgrounds and have varied personalities. Over the years it takes to acquire a medical education, there is a sifting of these diverse personalities into the different specialties.

The people who end up in each specialty often have similar characteristics that help define their reason for selecting that particular area of medical specialization. It has often been noted that those who end up in surgical fields tend to be more aggressive but also less empathetic to the feelings of others. Solutions to those who end up in surgical specialties are often much more black and white that to those in the medical specialties. "When in doubt, cut it out" is a simplistic rhyme that is used to describe the mindset of many surgeons. Those who head for internal medicine fields are often more intellectual and cerebral than those who opt for surgical areas. The joy of practicing medicine for those who choose to become internists is often contained in the excitement of learning a new fact or making a new discovery. Sometimes to an internist the diagnosis is far more interesting than the treatment. There are certain hierarchies of intellectualism that seem to occur in internal medicine subspecialties, but these seem to be more based on technology than on supportive care.

Family practitioners are seen as the physicians who are most likely to have the interests of their patients at heart. People who choose this specialty enjoy supporting their patients through hard times. Holding hands and a good bedside manner are often more important than the hard and cold facts of a disease or its cause.

A subspecialist may need to be called when the generalist's usual approach does not seem to be working, but the warm-hearted approach of these doctors can frequently cure some difficult and puzzling medical problems.

People who choose pathology like puzzles and difficult problems, but they are often uncomfortable around other people. They choose this field because it allows them to use surgical and internal medicine-thinking skills, but does not force them to sit with sick people and provide comfort. To a pathologist, such supportive care is often difficult and uncomfortable.

The person who selects pediatrics must combine features characteristic of a family practitioner with those of an internist. He or she not only has to deal with children and appreciate the differences between children and adults, but must also be able to explain facts and ideas to frightened parents. A pediatrician must have outstanding people and communication skills. Pediatricians rarely have to deal with issues of death and dying. As a group, they tend to choose this field because such issues make them uncomfortable.

The general pediatrician loves newborn babies and the excitement of the beginning of a new life. A pediatric oncologist is to some extent a totally unique individual. Such a person heads into pediatrics because of the desire to be involved in the formation and development of a new personality. Yet as doctors dealing with cancer in children, pediatric oncologists require a more realistic view of death and dying. They also must have the ability to deal with the intense emotions of the parents, child, and extended family as they try to cope with a diagnosis of a potentially fatal disease. Many in this subspecialty retain the innate fear of dying and death that tends to characterize those who choose pediatrics as their life work. Few people are able to combine the necessary personality traits and skills in order to work successfully in this field.

Some who end up as pediatric oncologists do so because they love the intellectual challenge that the diagnosis and treatment of cancer in children presents. In that way, they are very much like internists. Many of these pediatric oncologists spend their careers in university settings studying patients but not truly interacting with them on an emotional level. Some spend time in the clinical care of the children, but often leave most of the intense day-to-day work to residents and interns. Others find the stress and pressure too great and find a way to escape from the clinical setting as time passes. The burnout rate among people who have chosen pediatric oncology as their specialty is very high. Few are those who remain actively involved in patient care for their entire career.

For many years pediatric oncology was part and parcel of the pediatric programs at most medical schools. Even those pediatric oncologists who claimed to be in private practice did so in association with residency programs and all of the typical status items that are usually associated with being part of a university department. In the past 10 years, however, pediatric oncology has begun to move out of the ivory towers of the university into the private world. This privatization of childhood cancer care has come about as a result of major therapeutic advances. As a result most of the more common childhood malignancies now have fairly standardized and accepted treatments.

Economic realities forced upon the medical world by insurance companies and government medical programs have also provided the impetus to the movement of pediatric oncology into the private community. A third reason is that parents have become much more medically educated. There are increased demands by parents and by patients for patient-oriented treatments. The days when children with cancer served merely as tools to educate residents or to test new therapies seem to be nearing an end. The goals of pediatric oncology programs today must not only include education and research, but must also include patient care. The child no longer can be reduced to the disease or disorder he or she has. The overall needs, hopes, and aspirations of the child and his or her family must be taken into account.

In the 1950's and 1960's, the goal of pediatric oncologists was to find a way to produce remissions and extend the survival of children with cancer by a few weeks, months, or even years. Over the years since then the success of the therapies has been phenomenal. Almost 70% of children diagnosed with some sort of cancer this year can be expected to be cured. Some types of cancer produce substantially better outcomes. There are still some childhood malignancies that do not respond as well to our current therapies but newer strategies and treatments are constantly being developed. No longer are pediatric oncologists satisfied with getting a cancer to respond to therapy. The goal is to achieve a cure.

The definition of cure has changed also. When we first became able to cure some of these cancers, we thought little of what happened to the children years later. We found out that many of the treatments had in some cases resulted in unacceptable toxicity. The definition of cure now includes *the reintegration of the child into society as a productive member.* This means that pediatric oncologists not only must know the treatments and their side effects, but must also be aware of the developmental, social, emotional, physical and intellectual impact of the treatment of cancer on the children.

The stresses placed upon the pediatric oncologist today are greater than ever before. Despite the inherent difficulties in providing this all-encompassing care, the benefits of such total involvement in the life of child are great. A pediatric oncologist has the ability to make a profound impact on the life of the child for whom he or she is responsible. I do not believe that any other field of medicine allows and even demands that the doctor become so completely involved with his or her patients. I often wonder whether my colleagues who deal with adults with cancer feel the same intense emotional rapport with their patients that I feel with mine. When they do not seem to do so, I feel that they are missing out on something truly unique and special. It is highly possible that the much larger volume of adults who have cancer makes such intensity possible. Regardless of the field selected or the reasons for selecting that field, the finest physicians are those who are able to transcend their own personal needs and place their patients first. These transcendent physicians are the ultimate caregivers. They are physicians who are cognizant that a person's illness must be placed in the context of how that person relates to his or her environment. These special doctors help their patients cope with the changes that illness necessarily brings. Transcendent physicians are active listeners who always have their patients' best interests at heart. Despite all of the lists of best doctors and best hospitals that have been published by various interest groups, there are very few transcendent physicians. Most doctors I know are caring individuals, but few ever rise above the mundane to enter the world of true altruism and medical ministering.

Nowadays, with all of the changes occurring in medical financing and technology, I see even less selflessness. One of the few areas remaining where I believe one can find truly transcendent physicians is in hospice. Prior to the technological revolution in medicine, which started with World War II, death was not an event to be feared. Life had a definite beginning and end. Each was celebrated for the natural and awe-inspiring event that each was. Somehow, due to the amazing technological advances of the past fifty years, we have come to believe that people no longer need to die from disease. Even though the inevitability of death has not changed for a single human being, there is often a feeling that one must have an explanation for the death of a young person. The worst situation is one in which the parents, the doctors, the relatives, the friends, or even outsiders feel the need to assign blame to a death for which no explanation is adequate. As we have become more successful at treating cancer in children, we have become equally less accepting that children still sometimes die of that disease. This is in spite of the fact that cancer remains the second most common cause of death in children less than fifteen years of age in this country.

Hospice is a concept that embraces the reality of death. Hospice preaches that dignity and love survive even if the body does not. People who work in the hospice field believe that it is important to provide peace and support to the dying person. When it comes to a dying child, the need is often greater because the child is often unable to ask for him or herself. It is often very difficult for a father or a mother to admit that his or her child has reached the limits of current medical technology. Despite all efforts, their child will die. *Acceptance of the impending death and attempts to make it as peaceful, painless, and dignified as possible are the major goals of the hospice team.*

Participating in hospice requires enormous courage on the part of the parents, the child, his or her immediate and extended family and the medical team. It also requires a transcendent physician who can put the comfort of the child first and foremost. When I first told Marian of my interest in hospice, she told me that she thought that I must be deficient in some sort of vitamin. She asked me if I had some sort of death fetish. Once she obtained a chance to help me with a child in a hospice situation, she came to understand how life affirming and beautiful such an experience could be. Although I had learned about death and dying in children with cancer during my fellowship training, I did not truly understand either the hospice movement or the reasons for providing hospice care until my active duty stint with the Air Force. I had just completed my first year of active duty service and was feeling fairly secure in my abilities as a pediatric oncologist. One quiet afternoon while making rounds and teaching, I was called to my office to meet with a fellow military officer. This officer had spent much of his career in the Air Force and had been transferred to San Antonio only a few months earlier. He was not in the medical service like I was and so his bearing and mindset were much more military in nature. He told me that his son, Gregory, was 10 years old and had been diagnosed with a brain tumor two years earlier.

Gregory had initially responded to the radiation therapy that had been given at that time, but he was now having some new symptoms. His father was concerned that these new symptoms were signaling the return of the tumor. He asked me if I would evaluate his child. I readily agreed. The next morning Gregory was waiting in my office when I arrived at the Air Force base office. He was a very thin but bright young man who had such severe dizziness that he could no longer walk. He was seated in a wheel chair but even there he was leaning to the left side because he could not sit up straight. Sometimes he would slip down in his seat. When he slumped over, his father would stand and gently lift him to a more comfortable position. Further examination showed that he had significant left-sided weakness that extended from his face all the way to his leg. When he smiled, which was not often, the left side of his face did not move well. This created a crooked and one-sided smile that drew even more attention to his weakness. At first he would not talk and was withdrawn. After a little bit of time had passed, he began to be a bit more confident. Our conversation became more animated when we started to talk about baseball. He was an avid baseball fan and had loved to play when he had been well. Talking about his favorite game allowed him to warm up to me rather quickly.

Over the next three days X-ray studies were obtained of Gregory's brain. Gregory's father had unfortunately been correct. The tumor was much larger than it had been just a few months earlier. Gregory's father declined any further therapies and requested that Gregory be allowed to remain at home until he passed away. I had encountered little experience with hospice in my earlier training and none in my time in the Air Force, but I took a deep breath and said that I would try. Something inside of me told me that it was the right thing to do. I promised to try to provide Gregory with as much peace and comfort at home as I could. I first went to the administrators of the Air Force Hospital to check into various issues. I needed to verify that helping this family in this way would not be contrary to any Air Force regulations. I was somewhat surprised but pleased to find virtually no opposition to my requests.

Over the years that have passed since I first became involved with Gregory, I have discovered that those families who have a realistic and honest view of their child' s illness are the ones who are the easiest and most enjoyable with which to work. Such parents also tend to recognize and grasp the dilemmas of medical care especially during the terminal phases of a disease. This may be one of the reasons why hospice has proven to be such a purifying experience for me. In order for a family to be ready to undertake hospice, they must first have come to grips with the reality of their child's cancer and the fact that further therapy is unlikely to change the ultimate outcome. To reach this realization requires a great deal of painful soul searching. Many families have later told me that once they agreed to have their child placed into hospice, they experienced a sense of relief and peace knowing that their child would soon be released from the painful physical state which had caused him or her so much suffering.

Sometimes parents reach this state of acceptance before I do. When that happens, I must struggle with my own feelings that perhaps there still were some medical options that were worth trying. Other times I reach the realization that further treatment will be futile before the family does. That can lead to feelings of regret that the child must suffer through further side effects for very little benefit except to the family's need to retain some hope that a medical miracle might still occur. My belief is that medical miracles that do occur at such times happen in spite of and not because of the treatments which are being used. Concluding that there is little hope that conventional medical techniques will still produce a cure does not eliminate all hope. It just means that these hopes must be based on more spiritual beliefs. Gregory's family had reached acceptance of the boy's impending death from the brain tumor before they had even walked into my office. Gregory was old enough to have formed fairly adult views of life and death. He knew that he was going to die. He was far less afraid of dying than his parents were of watching him die. It was his peace of mind and contentment that allowed his parents to proceed with such strength. Gregory viewed his dying as just another adventure. He was not concerned for himself, as he was sure that he was headed to a much better place. However, he was very sad and worried about his parents and sisters. He was afraid that they would not cope well with his death.

This belief has been one which I have encountered many times when dealing with dying teenagers. Gregory's two sisters were both older than he was. They were both teenagers. The teen years are difficult because they are a period of time when one is trying to deal with issues of independence and self-realization. Teenagers rarely explore issues relating to their own frailty or mortality. They often have difficulties moving beyond their own needs and desires. With Gregory dying in the home, his sisters were forced to confront issues that even many adults find baffling and confusing. I was fortunate to find an excellent counselor who worked with them and helped them cope before and after their brother's death.

Following our initial encounter, I would make a home visit to see the lad about once a week. Never having done this before, I found the visits to be strange. I was not coming to offer any techniques to improve the child's clinical status. I was there to see if he had deteriorated further since my last visit and to reassure the parents that they were doing a good job in caring for their son. At the end of each visit I would review with Gregory's parents the changes which I had noted and give Gregory and his mother and father a big hug. Usually his sisters were at school when I came to the house. Reassurance worked both ways. They would thank me for coming to their house and let me know how much they appreciated what I was doing for them. What they did not know is that I was definitely the one who received the greatest benefits.

One day I brought a nurse from the Air Force hospital with me to meet the family and to help them deal with some nursing issues with which I felt uncomfortable. The nurse who came with me was the nurse in charge of all of pediatrics for the hospital. Her interest and involvement in Gregory's care proved to be enormously helpful. Not only did she help with the family that day; her visit made her an avid supporter of the hospice concept. She later helped me develop pediatric hospice regulations for the entire Air Force.

On the day that the pediatric head nurse visited Gregory's home with me, the young man had reached a state where he was unresponsive to outside stimuli. He no longer talked nor smiled. It was clear to his parents, the nurse and me that the end was near. At 2:30 the next morning I was awakened from a sound sleep by a phone call. Gregory's father apologized for waking me but he said that Gregory had died peacefully just a few minutes before. I told him not to do anything until I got to their house.

I struggled to dress in the dark so that I would not wake up my family and drove out into the night. That night was not only dark, but a dense fog had rolled in. The thick, almost impenetrable fog made visibility extremely poor. I had to drive slowly and carefully, but, fortunately, there were very few other brave souls on the road early that morning. Although I could usually make the drive between our two homes in about 20 minutes, that morning it took me more than an hour. While I drove, my thoughts were on Gregory and what I would have to do once I arrived at his house. Despite the *mental rehearsal*, I was not truly certain how to proceed. When I arrived, I walked up the pathway to the front door and rang the bell. I did not have long to wait before Gregory's father answered and I stepped inside. The house seemed sad and somewhat empty, but it also contained a sense of peace. I hugged Gregory's parents and then walked into the bedroom where I had spent so much time over the past few weeks. The boy's father told me that just before his son had taken his last breath, he had opened his eyes one last time, fixed his gaze on his parents and then smiled. This had given the grief-stricken parents great satisfaction and peace for they knew that they had done the right thing for their son. I checked Gregory to make sure he had no heart rate and was not breathing and then noted the time. As I gazed upon the thin, pale body in front of me, I felt a great feeling of sadness. The feeling was very similar to how I had felt when I had looked at Bobby, the first child I had known who had died. I missed them both, but I knew that I was a far better person for having known them.

Gregory's father wrapped an arm around my shoulder and said, "Thank you for making this possible."

The next few hours passed in a blur. I had found out that the police who had jurisdiction in that area were the first people who needed to be called. This was so they could determine if there was any evidence of foul play that might require the involvement of the medical examiner. The policeman arrived with twenty minutes of my phone call. My presence and the child's obvious condition quickly dispelled any notion that foul play was involved. The policemen who came to the house were polite and did their jobs thoroughly and quickly. After they called the medical examiner and explained the situation, they made a few notes and then left. Their visit lasted less than fifteen minutes. Once they departed, the funeral home was contacted.

A few weeks before Gregory died, his parents had visited a local funeral home and made plans for the boy's funeral. While this was very difficult for them at the time, it would have been much more painful and difficult if they had waited until after he died. Within 30 minutes of contacting the funeral home, a hearse drove into the driveway of the home. The removal of the body from the home brought all of us to tears as the absolute reality of Gregory's death sank in. In a short time Gregory's parents and his sisters and I were alone with our personal thoughts and grief. I stayed only a few minutes after the funeral home workers left. There seemed to be little that needed to be said. The morning that Gregory died was my 30th birthday. I did not celebrate it officially until a few days later but the celebration was less important than what had happened to me that morning. I felt that my experience with Gregory and his family taught me *what being a doctor truly meant.*

That initial hospice experience was unique, special, and almost overwhelming. While I could understand the need that Gregory's parents had to keep him at home, I had some difficulty understanding and appreciating the emotions attached. It seemed that what had happened was right and good, but I did not know why.

My next hospice experience with Jay helped explain why. Jay was 14 years old when I first met him. He had been undergoing treatment for a lymphoma, a malignancy of the lymph nodes that had been discovered in the front portion of his chest. Two years had passed since the malignancy was diagnosed. In that time he had received chemotherapy, radiation therapy, and two surgeries. His original pediatric oncologist had left the Air Force and so I had inherited Jay's care. Either because of or in spite of his treatments, the teenager had a keen sense of humor, an impatience with his treatments, and an amazingly mature sense of himself and his place in the world. Jay's father was an older man whose wife was several years younger. Jay was the oldest of three children. His younger siblings were just starting elementary school and his mother had recently found out that she was pregnant again. When I entered the picture, Jay was about to finish his therapy. He was looking forward to a life that included girls, football games and a full head of hair. Jay had been profoundly altered by his cancer experience. He was worldly and yet naive, knowledgeable and yet naive. He was an enjoyable combination of oxymorons.

One cold Friday morning I walked into my office. Jay had his chest X-ray taken that morning prior to receiving his last chemotherapy course. The X-rays had been a formality since I had no reason to suspect that there were any problems, but what the studies showed was a clear view of Jay's limited future. The lymphoma had seemingly recurred overnight. Sharing bad news is never easy. It was especially difficult that day since Jay was not ready to start treatment all over again. He also was definitely not ready to die or even face death head on. His reaction was marked anger. I certainly could not blame him. He had suffered through two years of nausea, hair loss, restrictions and pain. Ultimately it had been of little benefit. After he had gotten his anger a little bit better under control, we explored the various treatment options and together decided on an intensive chemotherapy program. Jay's mother had significant ambivalent feelings about starting all over again. She did not want Jay to have to suffer more than he was going to anyway. She had already accepted the reality of her son's illness and knew that further therapy was unlikely to make a difference in his ultimate outcome. Jay's father did not even entertain the thought that further therapy would not be given. He had the utmost confidence in the chemotherapy.

Still, despite their basic philosophical differences about the value of further chemotherapy, the two parents left the ultimate decision up to Jay. Jay knew that the odds that his tumor would respond to the chemotherapy were remote. He also knew that even if the tumor shrank, his chances that shrinkage of the tumor would lead to cure were even smaller. Despite this grim knowledge he was not yet ready to accept that reality. He decided to try a new combination of chemotherapy. Soon the medicines were flowing into his veins. It took only a few more days before he began to run fevers and vomit. The ordeal his mother had anticipated had begun. Jay was admitted to the hospital. Three days passed. Jay was showing few signs of improvement. When I entered his hospital room on the third day, his mother took me aside.

She held my arm as she whispered, "Dr. Lazarus, I know that my husband and my son think that a miracle is somehow going to happen, but I am more down to earth than they are. I don't know much about medicine, but I do know that I am not going to see any miracle other than the birth of this baby that I am carrying. Is there any way that Jay could be allowed to come home to die?"

"What about Jay and your husband?" I asked, "They clearly are not ready for that."

She honestly replied, "Surely we can think of something to allow them to continue to believe in their miracle. But what we are doing to Jay is wrong. I don't want him to die, but he is going to whether I want him to or not. Can't he be at home where we can love him best?"

Her words struck home. Just like when Gregory's father had let me know that he knew that Gregory was going to die from his brain tumor, Jay's mother had succinctly described my own feelings. I knew that she was right. I promised to make every effort to accomplish what she desired. Jay began to recover from the chemotherapy-induced problems four days after my talk with his mother. He was excited about going home. When we finally had some time alone, I asked him what he thought about the recurrence of the tumor and what he wanted for his future. He was more aware of the gravity of his situation than I had realized. He was very sad that he would be leaving his parents, sisters and unborn baby sibling behind. He was even more disappointed that he had nothing to leave behind for his soon-to-be-born brother or sister. He did not want his unborn sibling to grow up and not know that he or she had once had a big brother. He wanted to leave behind a *legacy* to show that his life had represented some meaning.

With some support of a sympathetic psychologist, we arranged for him to make a *videotape*. On the tape he told his new brother or sister what sort of person he had been. The taping was heartwarming and beautiful. When the taping was completed, he was at peace. He had accepted his fate and no longer needed or wanted further chemotherapy. He wanted to spend as much time enjoying his family as he possibly could. Jay's father had not reached the same emotional peace of mind achieved by his wife and son.

One week after Jay returned home, I went to his house to check on him. His father was with him. His father took me aside at the end of my visit and asked when further chemotherapy would be given. I told him that I could not start the chemotherapy until the boy's white count improved. Jay's blood count never did recover to an acceptable level after that initial course of chemotherapy so what I told his father was true. As the days home turned into weeks and Jay's condition slowly but steadily deteriorated, his father's question as to when we would restart chemotherapy was asked less frequently. Still, he seemed to accept the same explanation each time without complaints or questions. I think this allowed him to cope with his child's physical deterioration without having to deal emotionally with the reality of his son's imminent death. About three days before Jay died, I told his father that Jay was not going to be receiving any more chemotherapy.

His father responded, "I am so relieved! He can't handle any more and neither can I!"

Jay died peacefully on a Thursday morning. His mother called me at my office when he died and I went to his house as soon as possible. This time I was much better prepared than I had been when Gregory had died at home. Jay's family was quietly sad but also relieved. They knew that they had done what was best for their beloved son and brother. In an amazing coincidence, Jay's sister, Jennifer, was born that same afternoon. Jay had left his taped legacy for the sister he would never know. Her birthday will always be for Jay's family a day to celebrate and a day to grieve.

The peace, tranquility and love inspired by the hospice experience were now obvious to me. Several people at the Air Force Base had the opportunity to witness and even to participate in my experiences with Gregory and with Jay. Several nurses had helped in Jay's care, as had a social worker, a chaplain and a psychologist. They all felt a need to do more because they had been so profoundly moved by their involvement. I arranged a meeting of people I felt would be interested in planning a more formal hospice program. I wanted to establish formal regulations for running a pediatric hospice so that the program could continue even if its original founders moved away. In a short time we had crystallized our thoughts into guidelines.

The hospice guidelines we developed proved to be quite helpful, but we still had a few valuable lessons to learn from some of the earliest participants. Rebekkah was a 15 years old. I was asked to see her shortly after a large malignant tumor was found in her right hip. Rebekkah had complained of worsening pain in her hip for several months before her father, who was a radiologist, had obtained an X-ray. Within a day of the X-ray, she was in the office of the Air Force orthopedic surgeon. That orthopedic surgeon biopsied the tumor and called me once the diagnosis had been confirmed. He reviewed the girl's medical history with me and then added that the family was Old World. I did not understand what he meant be Old World. He explained that the father was the ruler of the family. He was a strict disciplinarian and insisted that his daughter not be told her diagnosis.

There are several points of view about *whether children should be told that they have cancer*. In the early days of treatment when outcomes were poor, the prevailing opinion was that children should not be told that they had a malignancy. It was felt that being open and honest with the children placed too much pressure on them and was too depressing. This is no longer the prevailing opinion. In fact, this belief is quite out of favor. Evidence now clearly shows that when a child is not told that he or she has cancer, there are significant difficulties with communication. Keeping secrets not only requires that large amount of energy be spent by the parents and by the medical staff to keep the child from learning his or her diagnosis, but builds up a wall between the medical staff and the child. The doctor-patient relationship is changed significantly by not informing the young person why he or she is receiving various treatments. Instead of being a caring and sharing interaction, it becomes a relationship where the doctor acts as the benevolent father (or mother) overseeing the care of a person who is incapable of making decisions for him or herself.

Recent changes in obtained *informed consent* have made Rebekkah's situation moot. If a child is felt to be old enough to understand his or her disease and the reasons for treatment, then he or she is required to give *assent to treatment.*

Assent is different from *consent.* Only parents, guardians and adults can give consent. Assent means that the child agrees to undergo the proposed therapy. In order to give assent the child must be given adequate information about his or her disease and the treatment that he or she will receive. At the time I met Rebekkah, disclosure of cancer information to the child was not mandated like it is now. Because I had not been out of my fellowship for long and did not want to irritate anyone, especially parents and other doctors, I agreed to withhold the diagnosis from the girl. This was quite difficult for me. I did not like secrets for they made me feel like I was speaking to the child from behind a tall barrier. It was even more difficult since Rebekkah's cancer had already spread into her lungs by the time it was found. Despite the ethical dilemma in which I found myself, the cancer responded very well to chemotherapy. Within a few weeks Rebekkah's hip was no longer aching and she was walking without pain. Six weeks after chemotherapy began, Rebekkah was due to receive radiation therapy to those areas of her body which had contained cancer cells at the time of the original diagnosis. The first six weeks of chemotherapy passed quickly and without incident. After examining the teenager in my office, I sent her to another building where the radiation therapist worked. The therapist measured the girl's hips and lungs and made marks with a magic marker on her skin so that the same spots could be irradiated each day. The initial session with the radiation therapist took several hours. Rebekkah dutifully went along with the time consuming procedure. The next day when she walked into my office, she had a puzzled look on her face.

"Dr. Lazarus, why are they going to give radiation to my lungs when my problem is in my hip?" she asked.

I had known all along that Rebekkah would eventually ask such a question. The only way to answer her was to tell her the truth. I told her I would answer her question but first I sent her to the nursing station to have her weight taken along with a temperature and blood pressure.

I then turned to her mother who had stayed behind and said, "I cannot continue this charade. The only way to explain why she is getting radiation to her lungs is to tell her that the tumor has spread into her chest. I plan to tell her what is going on with her body. I just will not use the word, 'cancer'."

Her mother did not argue. She just nodded her acknowledgment. When Rebekkah returned from the nursing station, I was in a bit of a quandary as how best to proceed. Rebekkah was a sweet, innocent, sheltered teenager who had always relied on her parents to watch out for her best interests. She lived in a world where she could not imagine her parents possibly doing something that was not for her benefit. I needed to answer her simple question honestly but I also needed to protect her faith in her parents. I told Rebekkah that the growth in her hip was called a tumor. I explained that a tumor was a collection of cells that did not belong where they had decided to grow. I then said that some of the cells from her tumor had broken off from the main bunch of cells and had spread to her lungs where they had started growing. Finally, I told her that the radiation therapy and the chemotherapy were being used to stop those cells from spreading even further. Rebekkah had few questions. I am sure that most 15-year olds have heard the words, "tumor," "radiation therapy" and "chemotherapy" and know that if they apply to something in their own body, then they must have some sort of cancer. Still, if Rebekkah now did know that she had cancer, she did not show it. Her face remained impassive and untroubled.

The next year passed quickly. Rebekkah needed to be seen frequently and we developed a close relationship. After the first few months had passed, she began to make fun of the way I said, "Wonderful." I would drag it out for an extra two or three syllables and she thought that the way I said it was hilarious. "Wonderful" became our code word. The word was used several times during any conversation. "Wonderful" was always guaranteed to bring a smile and some sort of joke. After 14 months of pain-free happiness, reality struck home. The pain in her hip returned and so did the tumor. Within one week of the onset of the new symptoms, she could no longer walk. A new intensive chemotherapy regimen was started, but the chances for cure had vanished with the relapse. After a brief period of improvement, the tumor again began to grow.

Rebekkah belonged to a religious Catholic family. After exhausting the available standard and even experimental medical treatments, there was little further that I had to offer. The parents suggested that faith might help where medications could not and they requested help in travelling to the Shrine at Lourdes where it has been reported that very sick people have had their illnesses miraculously healed. It took a few weeks and many phone calls to arrange, but at last the family was on their way to France. The results of their search for healing through faith were similar to the results for those children who have traveled to Disney World for a Make-A-Wish trip. The family returned refreshed and renewed, but the tumor was unaffected by the visit to the shrine.

Rebekkah's father steadfastly refused to discuss his child's condition. Shortly after I had first met him, he had told me that he had watched helplessly as his parents had died of cancer in miserable pain. He could not bear to think that his daughter would die of the same horrible disease and that he would have to watch her suffering and then have to bury her too. It was easier for him not to discuss the reality of Rebekkah's cancer than to deal with the crushing pain of losing his beloved child. Because of his need to maintain denial, most of the communications regarding the dying teenager were handled with Rebekkah's mother. She was a loyal and devoted mother and wife who had stayed home to care for the home and the couple's two children throughout their entire marriage. Like many mothers faced with the untenable situation of watching their child die, she was much more honest and realistic about her daughter's condition than her husband was. She asked me if her child could spend her last remaining days at home with the family and I agreed to try. Rebekkah was to be the first patient for our fledgling hospice program. The family purchased a waterbed for Rebekkah since it helped to ease the teenager's growing hip and back pain. When she first came home, she was able to get out of bed and walk to the backyard. As a few days and weeks passed, she became weaker and thinner. Her appetite decreased and she lost interest in her once favorite activities. On one visit to her home she asked if she could get to meet my baby who was 7 months old. Marian and I planned a picnic and arranged for all the hospice members to bring a dish for the party. We brought the drinks, a ham and a turkey. The picnic was a great success. Rebekkah loved playing with the baby and the baby took readily to her. Rebekkah and her mother smiled for the first time in weeks. Her father was quiet as usual.

He continued to refuse to acknowledge the steady decline in his child's condition although it was painfully clear to everyone else in the home. By avoiding direct discussions about Rebekkah's cancer with her father, I felt that I was doing him a favor. By not being direct I was keeping him from having to deal overtly with the reality of her impending death. Still, I felt from my conversations with his wife that he understood that his daughter's death was inevitable and that our goal was to allow her to die with peace and dignity in the home. Unfortunately, I learned that my assumption was wrong in a rather difficult way. About one week after the picnic, I received an emergency call from Rebekkah's mother. Rebekkah had developed difficulty breathing and her mother had panicked. She had called 9-1-1 and the ambulance had just arrived at the house when she called me. I told her that there were no medals given for successfully completing hospice at home. The purpose of hospice is to give the family strength and support while trying to cope with the impending death of a loved one. If she preferred to have Rebekkah in the hospital, that was not a problem for me. I told her that I would meet the ambulance at the hospital emergency room. The ambulance beat me by only a few minutes. Rebekkah was in significant respiratory distress. She was gasping for air and crying with each painful inspiration. Her parents were confused and panic-stricken. Even though a family may have been told what changes they might expect as their child dies, there is no way for them to be truly prepared for the realities of a painful dying process. The frightened and miserable teenager had an oxygen mask strapped tightly to her face. The emergency technicians quickly started an intravenous line. Just before I rushed into the room where she had been brought by the ambulance, she was whisked away for a chest X-ray. I took that moment to take her father aside. I started to talk to him about his daughter's condition but had to stop when she was brought back. I grabbed her X-ray and went to the closest viewing box. Rebekkah's father was a radiologist so that I knew that her X-ray would speak volumes to him about her drastic state. The X-ray was devastating. Rebekkah's lungs were so filled with tumor and fluid that virtually no normal lung tissue could be seen. It was amazing that she was able to breathe at all.

I turned to her father as he gazed with horror at the sight of his daughter's X-ray and said, "I have no more treatments. This tumor is growing so fast and I have nothing left which will stop it. This tumor will kill your child. Please let me make her comfortable. But I beg you not to make me put her on a respirator and prolong her dying."

He blinked hard and started to speak, but he did not get a chance. The oxygen tank that was supplying his daughter with a little extra oxygen and allowing her to continue gasping for air suddenly ran empty. Within a few moments, Rebekkah stopped breathing. Now there was no choice. With no permission from the family to forego resuscitation, full cardiopulmonary resuscitation was instituted. Soon the dying child had a tube in her throat that was connected to an artificial respirator. The fluids and medicines used to restart her lungs and heart had already caused her face to swell. She opened her eyes slightly for a moment. Her pain-wracked face was filled with panic and fear. In order to help her cope with the changes, heavy sedation was ordered. Within minutes the pain medicines were administered. Her thin, pale body relaxed and she stopped fighting the respirator. As Rebekkah relaxed and stopped fighting, the situation became less intense. When things had calmed down, I had some time to talk with the teenager's scared parents. Again I told them that Rebekkah was going to die even though none of us wanted that to happen. I asked for permission to place a DNR on her chart. DNR stands for Do Not Resuscitate.

Modern medical technology has led to many difficult ethical crossroads. The heart and lungs can often be kept functioning for days, weeks, months or even years in a person who is otherwise dying from a severe trauma or a progressive disease. The ability to forestall death greatly exceeds medicine's ability to restore life. Just because we can keep someone's decaying body alive does not necessarily mean that is what should be done. The problem is that there is no consensus on how to determine who should be placed on mechanical ventilation. Sometimes the parents of a dying child have tried to have therapies withdrawn but have met resistance from the doctors and nurses involved in that child's care. Other times the parents insisted on continuing heroic measures in spite of opposition by the medical team.

Several celebrated court cases have tried to resolve the many issues involved, but multiple ethical issues remain. Most of the time the ultimate decision of how to proceed has been left to the parents and the family. When the person who requires resuscitation is a fully competent adult, that person may have left instructions to family members on how to proceed should such a catastrophic situation occur. By making his or her wishes known before such an event through documents such as a living will or an advanced directive, the family can make the very difficult decision whether to resuscitate or not knowing they are doing what their loved one desired. Legally, minors cannot make their wishes regarding resuscitation known since they are not considered by law to be competent to make such decisions. However, this situation is changing particularly for adolescents. Even if they do not have the legal right to do so, many teenagers let their families know how they feel. In

Rebekkah's case it was quite different. Her parents had refused to discuss the progression of her cancer with her. This had blocked any avenue she might have had to let her parents know how she felt about this issue. I explained to Rebekkah's father that resuscitation would only prolong Rebekkah's dying process. If her heart were to stop beating and medicines and other techniques were used to get it started again, she would only return to the exact same situation she was in before the resuscitation. The cancer would still be in her hip and her lungs and probably other places in her body. It would continue to grow and cause her further pain and suffering. Rebekkah's father became angry with me. He accused me of wanting Rebekkah to die.

"I would never agree not to proceed with treatment." He vehemently exclaimed, "Where there is life, there is hope!"

"But she is dying," I despondently answered.

"No, she is living," he angrily replied.

"No, she is alive and just barely that," I retorted.

I think that my youth and relative inexperience gave me an arrogance that I do not think I have when I deal with families in similar situations today. I still feel that prolongation of dying is unjustified, but I recognize more fully the very painful and raw emotions attached to the Do Not Resuscitate decision. Part of my anger over Rebekkah's father's adamant insistence that we proceed to use all the weapons available in our medical armamentarium even though we could not reverse his daughter's underlying condition was due to my lack of awareness that her father felt like this. I knew that it had been a major mistake not to have fully understood his beliefs prior to engaging in hospice. Even though Rebekkah's mother was well aware of her daughter's status and had overtly agreed with the hospice plans, she sided with her husband. In front of him she acted as if she had never realized that Rebekkah was declining. At that time I felt like she had betrayed me, but now I know that she had no choice as to her behavior.

Despite my belief that what her parents wanted us to do was wrong, I complied with their wishes. For two weeks Rebekkah stayed on the respirator. In order to keep her unaware of her circumstances and unafraid of her surroundings, she was never allowed to awaken from her drug-induced stupor. Those two weeks aged her parents and me. I realized then and I am well aware now that my beliefs are not always shared by everyone. I had to learn how to accommodate my beliefs to the parents' points of view when the two were in conflict. I also discovered that an intensive care unit is a violent place where love and compassion and comfort are not always the first or even the major priorities. An intensive care unit is a place where death is an enemy to be defeated. Death is rarely accepted as an inevitable outcome of a progressive disease process. There certainly is a place in medical care for such a unit, but when death does occur, it is greeted with anger, bitterness and guilt. It is difficult to achieve acceptance of a child's death in such an environment and acceptance is critical to achieving peace of mind. Being at home during the dying process allows the family to deal with the reality of the impending death in an honest way. This allows the family to move more easily into the grieving process that necessarily accompanies such a loss.

I did find out that Rebekkah knew that she had cancer within one month of her diagnosis. She had been aware all along what was happening to her and why. The day she told me privately that she had known she had cancer, she told me that she regretted not being able to talk to her parents about her feelings. She knew that she was not supposed to know that she had cancer. That her parents would not speak about the cancer and had forbidden all health care workers to mention it had only served to isolate her from her family and from us. When she had most needed her parents to listen and to understand her deepest feelings, she had been prevented from doing so. *I have never again allowed a family to keep me from open and honest communication of a diagnosis to a child.*

Even at fairly young ages, children are capable of understanding simple and, sometimes, even fairly sophisticated concepts about cancer. The truth may be painful, but ignoring the facts or refusing to acknowledge them can be even more so. Following our experience with Rebekkah and her father, the hospice team developed an agreement form. Before a child and family could enter into hospice, the parents had to sign that they understood that all appropriate medical remedies had been exhausted and that they wished to have their child at home for as long as possible. In turn, the hospice team agreed to provide support for the child and the family. We never regretted adding this simple agreement to the hospice program. Some of my favorite memories and experiences have occurred in the hospice setting. This is not to say that I enjoy watching children die. The death of a child is a painful and draining event. Still, the acceptance of the reality of death and dying by parents, child, and medical staff elevates all to the level of the angels.

We share moments and ourselves in ways that no one who has never been there could ever fully understand.

My experience with Victoria proved to be one of the finest and most meaningful hospice experiences for me. I am a still very close friend with her parents even though Victoria died several years ago. Victoria was one of the most beautiful young ladies I have ever had the pleasure to know. She had long brown hair that shone with the luster of good health and careful grooming. She had a face that could have launched a thousand ships if she had lived in the days of Homer. Her demure and innocent personality immediately drew in those around her and made her words more meaningful. She had a vision of the world that was gentle and belied the reality of what went on around her. She was blessed with a very loving, close-knit, religious family who protected and adored her. But she returned their love with a deep respect and love of her own so that it was an even exchange. I met her in the intensive care unit of a local hospital after a neurosurgeon had removed a highly malignant tumor from the back of her brain. That tumor caused headaches and dizziness and vomiting for several days before it was found and removed.

When I first saw her, she was hooked up to various monitors with a large white bandage wrapped around her head like a tight turban. Her parents sat at her bedside, nervous and afraid. Her mother sat on her right side and her father sat on her left side. Each held one of the girl's hands, but they did not speak to each other or to their daughter. Looking at the scene, I thought that she looked like a beautiful Indian princess asleep on her royal bed surrounded by her adoring subjects. After introducing myself, I escorted the two parents out of the room to an adjacent conference room so that we could discuss Victoria's tumor and what we needed to do about it. I knew that I would have to explain the information to Victoria later when she awoke. Her parents listened attentively to what I had to say and then asked if their whole family could be included in the discussions. When I agreed, I was not aware of how large and extensive were the roots of this close family.

We set up a time the next day when we could speak. At the appointed time the next day, a large conference room was filled with people all anxious to hear what I was going to do for their beloved

Victoria. I reviewed the situation for the entire family. I have never been one to back off from meeting with all of the relatives interested in a family member's well-being. If they are there and they care, then it can only help to have them fully informed. This family was bright and supportive. They quickly grasped the difficulties and realities of what lay ahead for Victoria. Victoria received the news of her tumor and the plans for chemotherapy and radiation therapy with amazing aplomb.

Her only question was, "When do we start?"

After we confirmed that the tumor had not spread from its original location, a central venous catheter was placed. We were now ready to begin with her treatment. The chemotherapy was tough on Victoria but she faced it with great courage. The radiation therapy proved to be even more difficult, but, again, she handled it well. As time passed, I came to know and to love Victoria and her family. They were funny, caring, warm people who always appreciated my efforts on behalf of their beautiful child.

One dreary February morning, one and one-half years after the original diagnosis, Victoria came into the office complaining of numbness that started at her left shoulder and went down her arm. Victoria's symptoms were bad enough that I admitted her to the hospital. I was able to get a CT scan scheduled for that afternoon. Her parents sat anxiously at her bedside when I returned from reviewing the films with the radiologist. The scene eerily resembled the one in the intensive care unit when I had first met the beautiful young lady. I walked over to Victoria's hospital bed and sat down near the head. I took her hand in mine.

"Victoria," I started in a gentle, quiet voice, "I need to tell you why your arm has been numb lately. I am sorry to tell you, but your tumor has grown back."

A stunned silence at first filled the room. Then Victoria began to cry out, "Why me? I don't want to die!"

I answered, "I know you don't, sweetheart, but none of us has control over that."

Victoria's parents were stunned. They asked for a few minutes alone with their daughter and I left the sorrow-laden room with a very heavy heart. Victoria and her family had become very special to me and

I felt horrible that I had been forced to give them such terrible news. About 20 minutes later I walked back into the room. Victoria had made a complete turnaround. Now she was smiling at me.

She said, "I was nominated for the Miss Teen Texas Pageant and that is coming up in two weeks. Can I still go? I've already bought my gown and I really want to go."

Now it was my turn to be surprised. I had not expected that to be her response to my terrible news.

"Of course, you can go," I replied, "I can't think of anyone who represents the best of Texas teenagers better than you. I couldn't imagine them holding the pageant if you were not in it."

She smiled and softly thanked me. Then she said, "I'm really not that afraid to die. I'll just bet that God has a special place in heaven for all the children who have died of cancer. I know that heaven is a place without pain and I can have my hair back and I won't have to wear this wig. Besides, I'll already know some of the children since I met them through you and we'll have a lot of fun together."

Her statement was amazing. I know that I could not have been as brave under the same circumstances. We spent the rest of the next two hours discussing what options remained for further treatment. We decided to wait to start any further therapy until the pageant was over. Two weeks later she headed off to join in the pageant festivities. I asked if she were going to tell the judges about her cancer experience or that she wore a wig. Her answer was vintage Victoria.

"No, I won't tell them. Then they would just feel sorry for me and I would never know how I would have done just by being me. I just hope that my wig does not come off while I'm on stage because then they would definitely know."

I smiled at her. "How about if you take your wig off when they put the crown on your head as the winner?"

We both laughed when we thought about the reaction it would get from the crowd. The pageant was held in a nearby resort. Victoria and her family were gone for nearly a week. The day after the pageant ended, Victoria returned to my office. I had been unable to talk with her family for the entire week and I was anxious to know the outcome.

"How did you do?" I asked as soon as I saw her.

"I was one of the youngest girls there, but I was still chosen as one of the top 30 girls out of more than 200," she said proudly. True to her word she had not told anyone about her cancer. Her mother brought in a small picture of Victoria at the pageant. She was wearing a beautiful evening gown. The pink satin and lace creation looked stunning. Victoria wore a dazzling smile and radiated happiness. I could not imagine anyone being more special than she.

"It was a tough weekend for Victoria," her mother told me. "Her left arm ached and she was very tired, but she had a great time. It was definitely worth it."

I still do not know how she could get up in front of all those people and perform so soon after being told that she was probably going to die, especially when the tumor was performing tricks with her body the whole time. Along with her pretty face and figure and her undeniable charm, her undying spirit is what made her so special. Despite the very poor prognosis, Victoria opted to try a new chemotherapy regimen. She had no trouble handling the effects of the regimen, but, unfortunately, the tumor continued to grow in spite of our efforts.

Victoria was not yet ready to throw in the towel and give up. But before entering into another intensive phase of treatment, she decided that she would like to go on a special trip. We enrolled her in the Make-A-Wish program and she chose to go on a Caribbean cruise. Victoria had two younger sisters. Her mother and her sisters loved to shop and so planning their wardrobe for the cruise was a major undertaking. Victoria might have had cancer and she might not have felt well, but she also truly loved to "shop till she dropped." Their discussions about what they purchased to take on their trip were amusing. Her father and brother's clothes barely filled half of one suitcase while Victoria carried three large valises just for herself. I examined her the day before they were to leave. We hugged each other several times before I let them leave my office. I was so excited for them. Two days later, I received a long-distance call from one of the many islands which dot the Caribbean. I had visions of all sorts of disasters that could have happened when my receptionist informed me of the site of origin of the call. I picked up the receiver with great trepidation fully expecting to hear that we were going to need to find some way to transport Victoria and her family back to the United States because of some catastrophic change in her condition.

Instead, her mother greeted me with a hearty, "We are doing fine. But, somehow, Victoria has managed to get herself bitten by a horse!"

"What?" I called out half in relief and half in surprise.

"Can you believe it?" responded her mother. "We travel halfway around the world for a good time and my daughter gets bitten by a horse. Don't you think she has suffered enough?"

I wanted to laugh at that, but her mother answered, "I'm serious. They have these cute horse-drawn carriages that line the streets here. I was trying to get a picture of the family standing next to one of the better-looking ones. It was such a pretty horse. It had a hat with flowers on its head with its ears sticking through the brim. Of all of us to be attacked by that nasty beast, wouldn't you know it would be Victoria? Now, what should we do about the horse bite?"

I had never dealt with a horse bite before so I did not know exactly what to do, but I was thrilled that the call was not due to some emergency. I suggested that they see the ship's doctor for care. Before I said good-bye, I told her to have a great time but to stay away from any more horses. The remainder of their cruise passed uneventfully.

A few weeks after they returned, they held a party at their house. Several of the families and children under my care were invited to swim in the family pool and enjoy a picnic. Although Victoria was not feeling well, she sat with us as we watched the other children swim while the parents sat around and talked. At one point she dropped a napkin on the ground.

She turned to Marian and said, "Could you please pick that up for me?"

Victoria had cancer but she was not an invalid. She just loved having people wait on her. Marian, however, was a strong believer in self-reliance.

She looked at Victoria and in a sweet voice said, "Your Majesty, Queen Victoria, I am sure that you can do that for yourself."

With that, a new nickname was born. Henceforth she would always be known as Queen Victoria. Despite the neurological changes that had already affected her daughter's body and our honest and open discussions about the absence of truly good options for treatment, Victoria's mother was not at a point where she could accept that her child was going to die. I held another session with just Victoria, her mother, her father and myself to discuss what should be done. Together the family decided that a bone marrow transplant was the treatment that offered her the best chance of survival. The purpose of this type of transplant would not be to change her diseased bone marrow for another person's healthy bone marrow since there was nothing wrong with Victoria's bone marrow.

In Victoria's case, the bone marrow would be used to salvage her from the toxic effects of very high doses of chemotherapy. Under normal circumstances these very high doses of chemotherapy could not be given to her since her bone marrow would never recover from their suppressive effects. Since the bone marrow for her transplant would be obtained and then set aside and frozen prior to the delivery of the chemotherapy, it would be spared from the side effects of the intensive doses of chemotherapy. I tried to talk Victoria and her mother out of the procedure since I felt that Victoria would suffer from the toxicity of the chemotherapy medicines and yet would still not have a reasonable chance to beat the brain tumor. Victoria and her mother were convinced otherwise and wanted to proceed. I made the arrangements and within two weeks she was admitted to a nearby hospital's bone marrow transplant unit to have her own bone marrow harvested.

A few days later, with her bone marrow safely stored away, Victoria began to receive the intensive doses of chemotherapy medicines. Within a few days her blood counts had plummeted to next to nothing and she became quite ill. Despite all her difficulties, Victoria's resolve to beat the cancer never waivered. Shortly after completing the chemotherapy, her frozen bone marrow was thawed out and infused back into her body. It took a few weeks for her bone marrow to start to grow and repopulate her now depleted bone marrow space. Slowly, but steadily, Victoria began to recover from the worst part of the transplant procedure. About six weeks after entering the bone marrow transplant unit, an MRI scan was obtained. All involved with Victoria's care were anxious to find out whether the chemotherapy had made any difference in the tumor growth. The results of the scan were irrefutable. The bone marrow transplant had not changed the tumor at all. It almost glared from the black-and-white MRI film and defied us to stop it. With the evidence of the MRI scan in front of them, the family was forced to accept the fact that conventional and even experimental therapies were not going to change Victoria's ultimate outcome. I convinced Victoria's parents that the best place for her now was at home.

The family lived relatively close to my office so it was fairly easy for me to stay actively involved in her care. A few of the nurses at the hospital who had worked with her through her bone marrow transplant experience had fallen in love with her and her family. They wanted to stay a part of the child's care even after she left the hospital. One of those nurses had recently left the transplant service to begin home health care nursing. It was a simple matter to hire that home health agency to provide support so that nurse could continue ministering to the family. A few other nurses joined in and we soon had a hospice program in place.

The first few weeks after she arrived home passed quietly and uneventfully. Slowly and gradually though Victoria began to lose her ability to get around and finally was confined to her bedroom. The only time she left her rented hospital bed was to go to the bathroom. Soon, even that trip proved too taxing. A portable toilet was placed at her bedside so that her bathroom breaks would be easier. As time passed she became more confused.

Once when Marian made a home visit, Victoria looked at her with a wrinkled brow and asked, "What are you doing here in my hotel room?"

She began to mix up day and night. One time, while eating dinner, she demanded to know why her mother would feed her spaghetti for breakfast. The delusions brought on by the tumor and the medicines used to control her pain were cute and harmless. Despite her advancing condition, family, friends and caring loved ones were always around to provide support. It was a sad home but a home that felt comfortable and warm. Finally Victoria became unable to respond to those around her. Medications were continued to keep her from feeling any pain or discomfort.

About two months after she had left the hospital for the final time, a large group of people had gathered in her small bedroom at her bedside. Schoolmates, family members, her original pediatrician, nurses and I stood in her room and reminisced about this special teenager and how she had touched our lives. Her mother said that she had always wanted her daughter to remain 13 years old forever since 13 had been such a special and wonderful year for her. She guessed that she had gotten her wish because Victoria's birthday was not until the next week, and she knew that her daughter would die before then. At one point during our reverie, I looked down at the still beautiful but unresponsive child. Helplessly, I let out a little laugh. Several people in the room turned to look at me with quizzical looks on their faces.

I pointed at the child lying still on the bed. "I can't help it," I said. "I can't believe that someone dressed her in a blue top and then put on a purple head ribbon. Queen Victoria never would have allowed herself to wear such clashing colors. Isn't there another ribbon or another blouse that can be found so that her colors match?"

Everyone laughed. All of us in that room knew that Victoria would have indeed been appalled if she could have seen how she had been dressed that evening. Some of the tension in the room was relieved by my humorous comment. People began talking about Victoria's love of shopping and how she liked to dress well. We took out the album of the pictures that had been taken at the Miss Teen Texas Pageant. We were once again reminded of this child's beauty and inner strength. As we reviewed her album, the rhythm of her breathing began to change. The space between her inspirations began to separate further and further from her expirations. Without a word spoken, we all turned towards her bed. Within a few minutes, her breathing stopped altogether. Several of those in the room, including myself, began to cry. I felt a terrible loss, but I also felt a special honor that I had been allowed to be a witness to this moving and awesome moment.

Another hospice experience that will always remain special to me was the one with Matthew. Matthew was a very talkative 4-year old who had the typical confidence that all 4-year olds seem to have. 4-year olds not only know everything, they know that they know everything. The only difference between a 4-year old and a 14-year old in that a

4-year old will occasionally listen to his or her parents. Matthew had bright, brown eyes and a natural charisma that attracted and influenced those around him.

Like Victoria, he had been diagnosed with a brain tumor. The issues related to his treatment were a bit different than those with Victoria because of his age. Giving a standard radiation dose to his brain might have caused him to have problems with intellectual development. As a result, I recommended to his parents that we add chemotherapy to a lower dose of radiation therapy to try to get the maximal benefits from each treatment while trying to minimize the side effects of both.

Matthew had three older brothers. The oldest was in college and the next was a senior in high school. His third brother was already in middle school. Matthew had come along just as his parents had been expecting to move onto a new phase of their lives, but he was not an "accident." He was very much loved and desired. He had brought the excitement and curiosity of a young child back into the household. Matthew's father was an investment manager at a local bank. His mother was a dental technician who was somewhat relieved to have been able to give up the working world for the hard work that comes to those who have chosen to be full-time mothers.

From the moment he was born, Matthew was special. Of all her children, Matthew's mother most felt that her youngest held a spark of divinity. She told me later that she had always believed that he was on loan to her from a benevolent God who wanted her family to know what true belief, contentment and peace were all about. Only a few days passed from the time the tumor was discovered until it was removed by the neurosurgeons. Within one week of surgery, therapy was begun with a dose of chemotherapy. He received one dose of the chemotherapy each week for eight weeks and at the same time underwent radiation therapy daily, Monday through Friday. The technicians at the radiation therapy center were amazed at how much Matthew was able to tolerate without complaint. No sedation, coercion or bribery was necessary.

Each day he would arrive at the center and run up to greet his favorite nurse. When his turn came, he would climb up onto the treatment table with only a little bit of help. Within a few minutes, he would be asleep. The radiation would be given without any difficulty and the next day he would return to repeat the process. Despite his compliance and lack of complaints or irritability, he did have trouble maintaining his weight during the radiation. His mother tried all sorts of inducements but nothing seemed to work. He basically refused to eat. Finally, Marian made him a generous offer. She would give him an action figure from one of the then-popular children's television shows, but only if he ate well for one entire week. This was the motivation he needed.

He not only did not lose weight the next week; he even gained one half a pound. Marian soon found out that the cost to keep Matthew gaining weight was fairly high since he would not eat unless he continued to receive a similar inducement each week. Our experience with Matthew's weight loss during radiation therapy has not been uncommon. Many children who receive radiation therapy, especially for brain tumors, have the same problem.

Treatment with radiation produces fatigue and a loss of appetite. With the loss of appetite often comes a decrease in taste sensation that further aggravates the loss of appetite. The radiation also increases the amount of calories the child needs just to maintain his or her weight. The combination of nausea, decreased appetite, increased energy needs and weight loss produces a downward spiral that can result in severe problems if not interrupted at some point. Various means of supplementation of the child's nutrition must often be used to reverse the situation.

I recall one 10-year old boy who received radiation therapy for treatment of a highly malignant brain tumor. Like Matthew he began to lose weight even though he was taking liquid nutrition supplements. Finally I had a special plastic tube placed from his nose to his stomach (a nasogastric tube) so that he could receive larger amounts of supplements than he was willing to take by mouth. The extra feedings were given at night while he was sleeping. He began to gain weight again and to feel stronger. After several weeks of these special feedings, his weight had nearly reached its original value. I told the boy that if his weight had reached the target level by the next visit, I would stop the special feeds and remove the tube from his nose. One week later he returned. I held my breath as he got up onto the scale. He had reached the desired goal although only by a few ounces. We were both quite pleased.

As he stepped off the scale, he grinned broadly and said, "I guess I won't be needing these anymore." He then reached into his back pockets and pulled out several large rocks. I laughed really hard. I said that regardless what he truly weighed when he did not have the rocks in his pants' pockets, such resourcefulness merited stopping the tube feedings. He never again needed outside support. Matthew did not require tube feedings, intravenous supplements nor rocks. All he needed was those action figures. With those as a motivation, he continued to eat adequately and maintain his weight.

Once the radiation therapy treatments had finished, Matthew started on a regular chemotherapy regimen. Although the medications were fairly intensive, the treatments were given to him as an outpatient. This gave us a great deal of time to get to know and appreciate Matthew and his family. Matthew's parents were both warm and loving individuals who were very bright. They had a marvelous sense of family and a strong grounding in basic human values. Matthew was just as special as his mother had told me. He was very bright but not in a precocious or obnoxious way. He had a way of looking at the world that managed to combine the innocence of youth with wisdom that was far beyond his years. He trusted those around him and inspired trust in all that spent time with him.

About 8 months after he started treatment, Matthew again began to complain of the same symptoms that had first brought him to my attention. I wish I knew why some children do 'terrific' with various therapies even when their parents are not compliant with care and why others relapse early even though everything that could be done has been done. The difficulty of not knowing who will be cured and who will die is one of the major causes of stress. Every visit contains a potential for recurrence.

It is impossible to know who will be cured and who will have to deal with the return of the cancer. As time goes on, our answers become only negative. By that, I mean if the tumor disappears or the leukemia goes into remission, then the only news that I can give the family regarding a change in their child's tumor status is that the tumor or leukemia has come back. There can never again be the elation of the tumor shrinking and disappearing or the leukemia going into remission. This feeling of always waiting for "the other boot to drop" creates a sense of anxiety and depression for even the strongest persons. Time can ease the burden but can never completely erase it.

Despite the news that Matthew's tumor had recurred, his parents were not greatly surprised. It was as if they had always anticipated that God would ask for their son's gentle soul to be returned some day before they were ready for that to happen. One week after the tumor relapse was confirmed, Matthew, his brothers, his mother and his father gathered in my office. I reviewed all of the treatment options that remained. I still harbored some hope for Matthew. I really was not ready to abandon the idea that a second treatment could produce a response. Still, I felt that I had a duty to let the family know that choosing no further therapy was one of their alternatives.

At the end of our discussion, Matthew's mother asked if the family could have some time alone to discuss the options and make a decision. I respected the parents not only for including their children in the discussion but for also including them in the decision-making process. They understood that whatever option was chosen would affect not only Matthew but also the entire family. Together they decided that Matthew would not receive any further therapy. They wanted him to be at home and be made as comfortable as possible for as long as possible. Marian and I decided that we would be the entire hospice team because we felt so close to Matthew's family.

The progression of Matthew's symptoms occurred rapidly. Still, his time at home was very special for his family. Matthew was surrounded by a warm, enveloping love that was unconditional. Few people, even if they live a long life, will ever know such contentment. Such is the beauty of hospice. It forces the family to stop saying that they will get around to priority items later. They must deal with what is important in their lives in the present. There may never be another time to say, "I love you" or "You are special." As with my sister-in-law, Bella, hospice and the imminence of her death forced me to say the things I felt then rather than waiting for another day or time. As a result of participating in hospice, one is left with sadness but not with guilt or regret.

For a few weeks prior to his death, Matthew was irritable. For some reason, he took most of his frustration and anger out on the brother closest to him in age. This brother was at an awkward age. He was just entering the teenage years and was trying to cope with Matthew's declining status as best he could. He was very attentive to Matthew's needs. Still, Matthew chose this brother to be the focus of his anger. The dying boy would tell his preteen brother that he loved everyone else in the family except him. This boy was very sensitive and he took Matthew's words to heart. He was very hurt but he tried hard not to react. As time passed, Matthew became less and less responsive to those around him. He stopped eating about ten days before his death. But then he rallied. About three days before his death he suddenly became more alert. It was clear that his anger had cleared. His irritability was replaced with a simple acceptance of his condition. He told his family, including the brother to whom earlier he had been so mean, how much he loved them. His calm, accepting spirit was healing and peace-giving.

Following that day, he showed no more irritability or demands. Matthew was at peace. He no longer struggled against the physical problems that had plagued him for weeks. His face was relaxed and calm as he lay in his bed. His parents, too, were at peace with their decision not to pursue further treatments. They had accepted their son's fate. Acceptance is a critically important component of hospice. Once the parents have come to terms with the horrible fact that their child is dying, then it becomes much easier for them to let go of the earthly body. The spirit of the child becomes a part of his or her loving survivors. Acceptance brings peace of mind and of spirit and thereby brings dignity, love, compassion and even beauty to dying. Matthew died in the glow of that peace. All who had been a part of the process and a witness to the love in the home were transformed and strengthened by it.

I hope that these stories about my hospice experiences do not give the impression that I welcome the death of a child. Nothing could be further from the truth. I hate to see a child suffer, whether from a procedure or from a cancer. My goal is to relieve pain as best as I can. It is just that sometimes, no matter how great the technology, or how spectacular the medical advances, or how much no one wants it to happen, children die of cancer or from the side-effects of the treatments.

No matter how well-trained and how prepared, no one is ever really ready for the death of a child. It is important to be honest with parents in the face of reality. Families should not be led to think that their child with advanced cancer will be cured when virtually every other child who has had that condition has died. On the other hand, miracles do happen. Walking that thin line of honesty without excessive pessimism or unrealistic optimism is difficult.

Pediatric oncologists tend to be very optimistic people. Even at very dark moments, they often will see a shred of sunshine. It is important that they present things in a way so as not to produce false hope. Treatment options must be presented in an honest way with the positives and negatives reviewed and shared as completely as possible. The child should play an active role in the discussion if he is able to do so in a meaningful way.

The responsibility for making the final decision, which ultimately lies in the hands of the parents, needs to be in concert with the physician so that the family does not suffer needless guilt should the child die. My work in hospice has made me realize that whenever death is inevitable or appears to be so, hospice is a peaceful and loving alternative to the hospital.

Bone Marrow

In the past ten to fifteen years, bone marrow transplantation as a technique to treat many malignant diseases increased dramatically. As a relatively new technique, it has had to prove itself as a worthy cancer-fighting tool with the medical community. Even more difficult has been to prove to insurers and managed care companies that paying for this high cost treatment is worth it.

Studies have now shown that bone marrow transplantation may be the best treatment for certain cancers. The pediatric oncology community has been more willing to embrace the technique because more children are making it through the procedure unscathed and because there is an increasing cure rate for certain diseases. This is due to better techniques for support of the patient undergoing such a procedure and to better pre-transplant preparation.

A bone marrow transplant is used for two purposes. In cases where certain cells in the bone marrow are defective or growing out of control, the bone marrow transplant is used to get rid of the malfunctioning cells and replace them with healthy cells. The other purpose of a bone marrow transplant is the one for which we used it for Victoria. The transplant is used to overcome one of the major problems associated with the use of chemotherapy or radiation therapy.

High doses of chemotherapy or radiation might eliminate the cancer, but the high doses damage the patient's bone marrow so badly that it could never recover on its own. A better term for this type of bone marrow transplant is *bone marrow salvage*. Bone marrow salvage rescues the child from the bone marrow destruction produced by the very powerful treatments used to eliminate any last traces of the cancer in his or her body. Bone marrow transplant treatments are very intense and usually very difficult. The child often becomes exceedingly ill from the procedure. Sometimes the treatment itself is responsible for the death of the patient. When it works, however, bone marrow transplantation is a valuable tool in the pediatric oncologist's armamentarium.

Bradley represents one of the best examples of bone marrow transplantation making the difference in the child's ultimate survival. Bradley was a beautiful little boy when I first met him. I do not mean beautiful in a physical sense since boys are not usually referred to as beautiful. Still, his flaming red hair, effervescent personality and amazing creativity quickly captivated me. He first entered my life in the middle of a hot summer more than five years ago. Bradley had been well until about one month previously when his parents noticed some small bruises popping up on his arms and legs. Since he was an active 3-year old, his parents did not question the bruises too much until he began to have nose and gum bleeding, fevers and listlessness. Despite their recognition that their child was sick, they were unprepared for the diagnosis of *acute promyelocytic leukemia*.

Acute promyelocytic leukemia is an unusual form of leukemia. It arises in cells that are destined to become the type of white blood cells that kill bacteria. The leukemia freezes those cells at an early stage of development. *Promyelocytes* are usually very easy to spot when viewed under a microscope because the cells contain large granules. These granules contain chemical substances which, when released into the blood stream on the death of the cells, can activate the entire clotting system. Once the clotting system is activated, it is difficult to stop. The protein factors necessary for clotting may then be used up and this can lead to excessive bleeding.

It was this excessive bleeding problem that produced Bradley's increased bruising. It is difficult to walk into a child's room and tell his or her parents that their child has leukemia. It was no different for me when I walked into Bradley's room. The atmosphere in his room that day was electric. When the word leukemia was finally used and the diagnosis confirmed, silence descended over the room like a funeral shroud. The only sounds for a few minutes after I made the announcement that Bradley had leukemia were the rhythmic sounds of Bradley's soft respirations as he slept and the beeping sound produced by the mechanical intravenous pump pushing fluids and medicines into his small veins. I finally broke the silence by reassuring the boy's parents that there was much I could and would do, but they continued their shocked silence. I told the family that I would talk with them at a later time. Once I had made sure that Bradley's various medical problems were addressed, I left the room.

The next day the atmosphere was different. Bradley's parents had an entire night to accept the fact that the toddler, indeed, had leukemia. They had not dreamed our meeting the day before. They were now ready to hear what I proposed to do to treat their child's disease.

Explaining therapy to parents involves making complicated treatments understandable. Parents are caught in the unenviable position of approving treatments that (they are told) can and will be toxic. The alternative to these powerful treatments is for their child to die of the disease. Many parents sometimes feel that they are in a no-win situation. With the increasing cure rate for childhood cancer as a result of these intensive therapies, the choice for therapy is often a very positive one.

It is important, however, not to scare the parents away by being too graphic about potential side effects. Decreasing the parent's fears over the potential side effects requires a combination doctor, educator, psychologist, stand-up comedian, and a person who can be a caring human being. Nothing in my medical school, residency or fellowship training prepared me how to combine all of these traits. My style has been created over the years by personal and professional experiences and by watching and observing other physicians. I try to adjust my presentation to the needs of each family and to the situation at hand. Mostly I try to treat the families according to the Golden Rule. I make every attempt to treat the family in the manner in which I would want my family to be treated should we ever find ourselves in a similar situation.

A physician's style is uniquely his or her own. Some are comfortable and caring, some clinical and authoritative, while others rely on humor. I feel that the time I spend with the parents and their child is the most important thing I can do as a physician. The amount of time I spend depends on the child, the disease, the ability of the parents to understand the information presented and how easily rapport is established.

I quickly found myself being drawn to Bradley's parents. Both were well-educated, interesting people who loved their child and only wanted the best for him. We talked at length about the toddler's disease and the planned treatment. We explored the options and reviewed the pros and cons of each in detail. Bradley slept through most of our conversation. Near the end, he opened his eyes and smiled at us with that absolute innocence only seen in young children. His mother picked him up and hugged him to her chest. He stuck his thumb in his mouth, nestled into a comfortable position and listened to the rest of our discussion with an intelligent look on his face.

When I had finished with what I wanted to cover and had answered all of the parent's questions, I turned to Bradley and said, "You are such a good boy. I know that you and I are going to be good friends."

Bradley did not respond. He continued to stare at me while he sucked on his thumb. As I stood up so did the boy's mother. She held him tightly with her right arm and hugged me with her left.

"We are going to fight as hard as we can. With God's help, we will win!" I whispered in her ear. I then turned to the boy's father and said, "You deserve a hug, too!" We clasped each other tightly. I then turned and left.

The next few days were filled with tests, discussions, questions and a lot of bonding. Soon, chemotherapy was started and Bradley's blood count began to respond. Other than a few fevers, Bradley never behaved as if he were sick. He was a delightful, happy child who always cooperated with examinations and procedures. This was unusual for a 3-year old, but this was an unusual and special 3-year old. Despite the intensive chemotherapy, Bradley's count did not go down as far as I had expected or hoped. I tried to keep up a brave front for his parents, but it became progressively more difficult with each passing day. One mother once told me that she could always tell how I felt by looking at me. She said that every emotion I felt was written on my face like a line in a book. I am sure that Bradley's parents could see my discomfort. I am sure that is why they were not shocked when I told them that their son had failed to go into remission with his first round of chemotherapy. We chose to try a second time, but, again, the results were the same. The malignant promyelocytic cells continued to sit in his bone marrow as if daring us to try something different.

After the second try at inducing a remission failed, I presented the options for further therapy as honestly as I could. In spite of two failed chemotherapy courses, Bradley was continuing to feel and look well. I offered the possibility of using different medications, but I did not feel that altering medication was the best course for their child. A hospital in a nearby city was testing a new agent that was looking extremely promising for this type of leukemia. I had also found out that Bradley's 11-month old sister completely matched her older brother. She represented the best option of all: a chance at a bone marrow transplant. I felt that the only chance that Bradley had to beat the leukemia was first to receive the experimental agent and then to undergo a bone marrow transplant using his sister's bone marrow cells. His parents agreed. It took me three days to make the arrangements with the hospital where I planned to send the boy. Two days later Bradley was on his way. His parents were optimistic about his chances for success but they were realistic about what they were facing. A week later they called me to let me know how things were proceeding. Within days of arriving at the new hospital, Bradley received the experimental medicine. It took only a few days for his blood count to improve. The plan was for him to be treated with the experimental agent for about three weeks before proceeding to the bone marrow transplant. However, one week after the experimental agent was started, a bone marrow examination showed that his leukemic cells had still not completely responded. Bone marrow transplantation was now his only option.

Bone marrow transplantation is performed by giving the patient very high doses of chemotherapy sometimes with whole body radiation. Giving the initial treatment usually takes 7 to 10 days. The patient is then allowed to rest for about 48 hours and then the bone marrow transplant is performed. The infusion of the bone marrow is actually an anti-climax. The bone marrow, which has been set aside for the transplant, is filtered to remove things other than bone marrow cells. Once cleaned by the filtration process, the bone marrow is then infused into the patient through the intravenous catheter. Sometimes, especially if the bone marrow was frozen before being used, the bone marrow is pushed into the patient in giant syringes. Otherwise, it is infused into the recipient just like a blood transfusion. It is following the return of the bone marrow that the difficult period starts. The medicines and radiation used to treat the original cancer take effect and the patient's own diseased bone marrow is destroyed. It takes 2 to 3 weeks for the bone marrow that was infused back into the patient to grow. During that 2 to 3 week period, the patient has very limited defenses. Multiple viral, bacterial and even fungal infections as well as terrible mouth and skin sores are commonplace. Many patients develop terrible diarrhea. In order to provide some protection, bone marrow transplant recipients are kept in a special unit where they can be protected and isolated. Even after the bone marrow has finally grown back, the patient remains at risk for unusual infections for a long time.

The removal of the bone marrow from the donor results in few problems for the donor. The donor is put under anesthesia because the multiple bone marrow punctures that are necessary are painful. Bone marrow cells regenerate themselves so the effects on the donor's blood count are temporary. The donor's hips are usually sore after the procedure because the marrow is harvested from the back of the hips.

One of the most difficult things for doctors, patients and families to realize is that despite all of the problems which a person goes through during a bone marrow transplant, there is still no guarantee that the cancer will be cured. Enduring a bone marrow transplant is never easy although some people have an easier time of it than others. It was very difficult for me to send Bradley's family off to another treatment program. I had to admit that my hospital and I had limitations in what we could offer. I feel that it is very important for a physician to be able to recognize and admit his or her limitations. When better or more effective therapies exist elsewhere, it is the duty of the patient's doctor to search them out and make them known to the patient. It is the patient's and family's responsibility to make a decision as to whether they wish to proceed with such a treatment. Parting with Bradley and his family was tough. I knew that the path on which they were headed was not an easy one. I also knew that the alternatives were worse.

Another thing I especially dislike about sending a patient off for treatment in another city or state is that I do not get to see them or even hear from them very often. Every now and then I may receive a phone call from the parents letting me know how their child is faring. More often they are so busy or anxious that they forget that I am waiting for them to return safely. Fortunately, Bradley was receiving care from a wonderful doctor. Every week he would send me a letter updating Bradley's progress. It was just like getting a letter from a child who has gone off to camp. I looked forward to each letter. Even if the letters were dry and somewhat lacking in emotion, I could read between the lines. Bradley went through the bone marrow transplant process as easily as he had gone through the initial unsuccessful therapy. Two months after I had sent the family away afraid I would never see the inquisitive red-haired toddler again, they returned to my office. We held a joyous reunion. Bradley looked and felt great. He had no hair and was wearing a special mask over his mouth to keep out germs, but he was the handsomest child I had ever seen (other than my own).

The months and years have passed quickly since that day. Bradley's red hair grew back and his mask is gone for good. His bone marrow, once filled only with malignant cells, is now normal-appearing. Bradley is once again a happy and playful child. What a special treat to know that I have played a role in this young man's life. Describing what it will be like for a child to go through bone marrow transplantation is like trying to describe what it will be like to ride a roller coaster to a person who has never seen an amusement park before. One could read about the ride and know how big the cars were or how fast they traveled, but that could only give the reader an idea of what to expect. Talking with a person who had already been on a roller-coaster ride might help a little bit because it would let the person know that it was possible to ride the roller-coaster and still survive. But there truly would be no adequate way for the veteran rider to describe the feelings that occurred to him or her before and during the ride. Thus one might learn more about the physical features of the ride but would not be able to fully grasp the psychological and emotional aspects associated with it. The only way to understand the rapid, dizzying rises and falls that occur while on a roller coaster is to actually get on the ride. The problem with that is that by the time one finds out that the ride is more scary than fun, it is too late to get off.

If asked now, Joshua's mother would probably say that bone marrow transplantation was no big deal. However, before her son went through the transplant, she needed 5 months of discussions, prayers and consultations to convince her that it was the right thing to do. Joshua was a handsome and very active 2-year old who first came to my attention several years ago when he was found to have leukemia cells in his blood stream when a routine blood count was obtained. His family practitioner sent him to my care. Despite his relative lack of symptoms, his bone marrow was found to be filled with leukemia cells. Joshua had acute myelogenous leukemia, a somewhat rarer type of leukemia in children but a much more difficult type to treat and cure. Joshua went into remission with ease, but I knew full well that his form of leukemia had a high risk of recurrence. I arranged to have some of Joshua's bone marrow frozen and stored once he was in remission so that he could undergo bone marrow transplantation at a later date. As the time for the procedure approached, Joshua's mother became more and more anxious. Discussing the idea of undergoing a bone marrow transplant and actually going through one are completely different. After several weeks and multiple in-depth discussions, she finally agreed to have Joshua proceed with the bone marrow transplantation. Joshua was soon admitted to the hospital for the treatment. Despite her fears about what might happen to her son, Joshua set a record for the shortest stay for a bone marrow transplant. Seventeen days after he entered the hospital, Joshua was well enough to leave.

The only major problem was boredom. During the period when his blood count was very low, he was not allowed to leave his room. He would quickly lose interest in the hundreds of toys that were haphazardly scattered all over the floor around his minimally-used hospital bed. There was only one day in the entire 17-day period that he complained of not feeling well. I wish that all children who went through bone marrow transplantation could have as benign a course as that experienced by Joshua. I do not often tell parents whose children are heading into bone marrow transplantation about Joshua's experience because it raises parents' expectations that their child will also have a trouble-free transplant. I saw Joshua and his mother just last week. Joshua has virtually no memory of the transplant he underwent more than 8 years ago. His mother, however, now thinks that transplantation is not a big deal.

Bubba had a much more severe course with many of the problems that can be seen with bone marrow transplantation. I first became aware of Bubba when he was 7 years old and found to have ALL. He was a cherubic child with a round, innocent face and wide, blue eyes. He had a fair complexion and blond hair that was lighter and finer than that of either of his parents. He was a combination of the best features of his attractive parents. For all of his winsome looks, he was a shy child. He was cautious with those who entered his life, but once he knew and trusted them, he gave his love and affection with all of the enthusiasm that only a child could muster. He was never rude with those who did not merit his affection. He merely gave them very little attention or time. He saved his love for those who were special to him. It took me some time before I was allowed within his inner circle. Marian did not need to wait. She achieved honored status almost from the instant the two met.

Bubba was very frightened of all the technology and treatments that went with having leukemia. For him the worst were the shots that he needed to get during the first month of his leukemia treatment. Marian understood his fear and helped him learn how to cope with it. She never made light of his anxiety. After the second injection, he decided that only Marian could give him the shot. Even if it meant waiting many minutes or even close to an hour, he would wait for her. He never cried in her able hands. The first few months of leukemia therapy were difficult for Bubba. He and his family were forced to make many changes. Somehow, as with most families, the unfamiliar and alien treatments soon became the routine of their lives. Soon things developed into a new but now normal routine. About 14 months after his leukemia was diagnosed, Bubba began to have problems with a low white blood cell count. When that happens and the child is on maintenance chemotherapy, it is most often related to the medications or to an infection. Most often the blood counts will improve in a few days to a few weeks after the medicines are stopped. Bubba's count, however, did not improve. After two weeks of waiting for the low counts to recover, I performed a bone marrow examination. The smear of the marrow was disheartening. The leukemia had recurred.

It is an extremely poor sign when the leukemia returns in the bone marrow while the child is still receiving chemotherapy. It is a clear sign to the doctor that the child's leukemia cells are resistant to the best medicines available for the treatment of leukemia. Most of the children who relapse so early will go on to die of the leukemia. However, some have been cured by bone marrow transplantation. Most of the cures after early relapses have occurred during a time when treatments for ALL were not very intensive. The newer treatments are more effective at producing a cure the first time around. However, when a patient relapses, they are much less likely to respond and be cured. It was a hot and sticky early August day when Bubba was admitted to the hospital to start a new course of chemotherapy. Before he could go for bone marrow transplantation, he had to achieve a second remission. During the first few days of the new therapy, long discussions were held with Bubba's parents regarding plans for a bone marrow transplant. The first thing we did was look for a potential match. Within one week of starting the new treatment, we knew that Bubba did not match his two younger sisters. His bone marrow transplantation could not be done without having an appropriately matched marrow.

Since Bubba had no match in his own family, we contacted the National Marrow Donor Program. The National Marrow Donor Program is a federally funded program in which people who volunteer to donate their bone marrow are registered. The people who volunteer their bone marrow give people who need bone marrow transplants but do not have a match a second chance. However, a bone marrow transplant using a matched relative is difficult enough. When the source of the bone marrow is unrelated to the recipient, then more problems can be expected. Despite knowing of the increased difficulties and greater danger, Bubba's parents felt that they had little choice but to proceed. Bubba did go into a second remission with the new therapy. While he was continuing to receive chemotherapy, a search was made for an appropriate volunteer donor. It took three months to find an acceptable donor.

In early December Bubba entered the hospital to start the preparative regimen for the bone marrow transplantation. It may seem somewhat cruel to start an intensive therapy such as a bone marrow transplant in the same month as Christmas. Leukemia, however, does not celebrate holidays nor does it recognize special occasions. The time to start such a treatment is when everything is in place and ready to go. Early December was the right time for Bubba.

During the first week of the hospitalization, Bubba was put through a thorough evaluation to make sure that his body could handle the intensive bone marrow transplant that was to come. A bone marrow examination was done just prior to starting the high-dose chemotherapy medications. Although the initial examination of the bone marrow looked like the leukemia was still under control, further testing showed that the leukemia cells had already started to grow back. This unfortunate news was not available at the time that Bubba started into the procedure. If it had been known that the leukemia was already returning, I am not sure that we would have chosen a different course. Bubba's options and alternatives were already severely limited. Still, the news that he was not in remission when he started the transplant suggested that his long-term survival was doomed from the outset.

The first two to three weeks of the transplant procedure passed quickly and quietly. Bubba did get a bit ill from the medications used to eliminate any residual leukemia cells from his body, but he retained his fighting spirit and enthusiasm. Around the fourth week he developed a rash that started around his neck but, within a few days, had covered his entire body. At first the rash resembled a severe sunburn, but then it began to darken. Bubba had developed *Graft vs. Host Disease* (GVHD).

GVHD is a problem unique to bone marrow transplantation. It is the opposite of the rejection that can occur with other organ transplants. When a person receives a kidney from a donor, the immune system of the recipient tries to get rid of the foreign kidney. Immune cells are sent to the new kidney to try to reject it. If medicines to suppress the recipient's immune system are not given, then the immune cells will be successful and the transplanted kidney will fail. In a bone marrow transplant, the immune system of the recipient is deliberately obliterated so that the new bone marrow cells will grow and develop. The immune cells of the donor (the graft) remain active once they grow in the new body. The problem is that these immune cells retain the characteristics of the donor and do not acquire the characteristics of the recipient (the host). As a result, once the immune cells of the donor grow back in the host, they sometimes reject the host. This can result in severe skin, lung and gastrointestinal problems. Sometimes the rejection is so severe that it can kill the host. GVHD tends to be more severe when the donor was not related to the recipient.

Bubba soon he looked like someone who has spent too many hours baking in the sun too long. Not long after the rash appeared, he developed other symptoms of GVHD. His temperature increased and he began to feel poorly. During the fourth week after receiving the marrow of a matched stranger, he rallied and began slowly to improve. Just when things started to look better, he developed pneumonia. Antibiotics and breathing treatments were added to his already impressive medical armamentarium. One day, about an hour after a breathing treatment, he began to cough and sputter. Suddenly blood poured out of his mouth as it spewed up from broken blood vessels in his lungs. His father, who had been sitting at his bedside, screamed out for a nurse. The nurse ran into the room, but stopped and stared in horror at the scene which confronted her. Bubba was having problems breathing. The blood pouring into his lung's air sacs and out of his mouth and nose was interfering with his ability to provide oxygen to his body. Amid all the chaos the nurse initially could not locate an oxygen tank or a mask, but finally one was found. The mask was strapped over the struggling child's mouth and oxygen began to flow into his tortured lungs. Some of the panic left his face, but he was still having difficulty breathing and blood was still flowing freely from his mouth.

As the situation calmed a bit, the nurse called in reinforcements. Within another 20 minutes he was rushed to the PICU where a tube was placed through his throat into his major airway so that a machine could do the breathing for him. The respirator not only allowed him to rest but increased pressure could be forced into his lungs to push the blood back into the blood vessels. Bubba's body finally relaxed as the respirator improved his lungs. His father was still shaken by the disaster that had befallen his child. A chest X-ray was obtained shortly after the boy was placed on the respirator. It showed that the bleeding had occurred throughout most of both lungs, which left the child with very little usable normal lung tissue. Still Bubba was a fighter and he continued to improve over the next 4 to 5 days. For several minutes after his lungs had started to bleed, Bubba had not had enough oxygen for his body. This lack of oxygen had damaged his liver. The boy's liver stopped processing a yellow pigment called *bilirubin*.

The bilirubin, which normally passes through the liver and into the gallbladder and intestines, began to back up into Bubba's blood stream. The excess yellow pigment was stored in his skin. Within a few days Bubba's skin had turned a deep yellow from the bilirubin which made him look like he had been lying in a tanning booth for a long time. On the fourth day after the lung-bleeding episode, Bubba had improved to the point that it was felt that he was ready to have the respirator removed. For the first hour after the tube was removed from his throat, he did well. But he was too weak and tired to sustain the effort needed for breathing, and he soon weakened. As his muscles fatigued, his oxygen level fell. Soon he became panic-stricken with a feeling that he was suffocating. It took less time to react this time, but, once again, his parents went through the intense and agonizing emotions of possibly seeing their child die. Within moments the airway tube had been reinserted and the respirator restarted. Once Bubba was again stable on the respirator, it was decided that he needed more time to heal and gain strength. Two weeks later he was again tried off the respirator. This time the attempt was successful.

Despite the improvement in his lungs, his problems continued. His liver worsened instead of improved. High fevers became the rule in spite of intensive searches to find their cause. The days passed slowly and agonizingly. Each moment Bubba might show some improvement or he might be worse. The process was not only miserable for the child, but it was a gut-wrenching tragedy for his parents. After three long and arduous months, his mother began to ask the doctor for just one thing— she wanted to have her child at home in his room for a brief period for one more time. She was beginning to realize that anything more was unrealistic. Mixed into her agony and pain was the fact that Bubba's grandfather had died of a blood disease just a few months earlier. The wounds left by that death were still fresh.

Despite promises that he might be able to go home for a while, Bubba would rally for a short while only to lose ground again just a short time later. His fighting spirit, so strong and confident a few months earlier, began to wane under the constancy of being ill and feeling bad.

Marian and I would make frequent visits to try to keep his morale up. Marian could always get a smile and a laugh from the desperately ill little boy even at his darkest moments. She would try to dance or sing which would amuse him. Despite her wonderful sense of humor and ability to see the positives even at the worst times, Marian remained very realistic and honest. She knew that Bubba was losing the fight and she joined with the boy's mother in the push to get him home even if it was just for a day or two.

One day when I entered Bubba's room, I noticed that he looked even worse than usual. He had a gray pallor that could be easily seen under his normal golden, bilirubin-induced color. He no longer responded to those around him. I sat down in the chair next to the very ill boy and touched his arm. His father sat on the other side of the child's bed. Few words were exchanged. The room felt restful but very sad. Without a warning Bubba turned his head toward his father and began to moan.

His father leaned in and asked, "What is it, Bubba?"

Another soft moan emanated from the child's dry and cracked lips.

"I love you, too!" his father answered. Those were Bubba's last words.

Shortly after my visit he was transferred back to the ICU and one again hooked up to a respirator. Dying is often not the neat and clean process that is shown on television or in the movies. It occurs at unpredictable times and in often painful and drawn-out ways. Marian and I might have been ready and we may have accepted the reality of what was happening to Bubba, but his parents had not. They still clung to tiny shreds of that elusive cloth known as hope. Somehow, they felt that Bubba would again overcome his horrible condition and rally. They had previously been told two or three times that he was going to die, but he had not. His parents retained their hopes that he would again triumph against overwhelming odds. For four days he was maintained on a respirator, too weak and exhausted to breathe on his own. Bubba had finally accepted the fact that the battle for life is not in how long one lives, but in how well one lives in the short time one is given. Bubba had given and received unconditional love during his brief tenure. He had lived a full and fulfilled life even though others might want to think about all that he might have done had he survived.

The truth is that such speculations do not change the fact that Bubba died. None of the dreams and hopes for his life will ever be realized, so he and we must be satisfied with all that he did accomplish in such few years. On the morning of the fifth day, a Sunday morning, Bubba's heart rate and blood pressure fell. With many loved ones at his bedside, his ordeal finally ended. The tears flowed freely, but with a certain sense of relief that this sweet and special boy had finally been released from his agony.

Pain Management

Many times I am asked how I could possibly work with children who are ill with cancer. People assume that it is morbid to be involved with children who may die. I see my occupation in a very different light. I know that I did not cause the cancer and I truly do not have the power to make it go away by myself.

Using the best treatments which have been developed by national and international leaders in my field, I know that many of these children will be cured of diseases that not too long ago were felt to be incurable. Some children, however, will not be cured and will eventually die of their disease. There are others who will suffer from the side effects of the intensive treatments and die or be damaged by them. If I can make the time these young ones have as meaningful and as pain-free as possible and if I can help the children and their parents and families cope better with the disease and its consequences, then I have made a difference in someone's life. I feel that the true goal of a medical doctor is to impact someone's life in a positive way. The world would be a better place if that were the goal of all people.

Despite my very positive outlook, it is terribly distressing and stressful to watch a child in pain. Pain control has become an extremely important part of what I do. Most of the children for whom I care have to endure multiple diagnostic tests such as bone marrow examinations, spinal taps, X-rays, MRI scans, CT scans, nuclear medicine tests, biopsies and surgeries. At best, these examinations are frightening and dehumanizing. At worst, they are painful and dangerous.

During the time I was completing my training, very few programs used any sort of sedation to help children cope with the various diagnostic and treatment procedures. I do not know if this was because the sedation might have increased the time it took to perform the studies or whether there was fear over potential side effects. Twenty years ago there were few safe sedatives available. In addition, our understanding of the mechanisms of action of these medications was not what it is today. Some child psychologists were trying to use hypnosis and other distraction techniques to help children get through difficult times, but for the most part their findings were ignored or looked upon as fairly unimportant since the overall goal was to cure the child. The child or parent's peace of mind and comfort were secondary to that goal. Pediatric oncologists were totally focused on finding ways to cure the various childhood cancers. The fact that the costs of cure were often exceptionally high was not a high priority. My experiences during my training helped shape my view that there was a need for better and more effective pain relief to help children cope with frightening or dangerous tests and procedures.

The memory of one child in particular stays with me to this day. Her experience convinced me that pain relief was an important part of my role as a pediatric oncologist and as a human being. Candy was a beautiful 4-year old girl with curly blonde hair and crystal blue eyes. Her diagnosis of ALL had been devastating to her and her family, but she had responded well to therapy. I do not recall how she handled the many necessary bone marrow studies, IV medications and spinal taps of the first few months of treatment. I do remember with crystal clarity, however, her reactions to procedures performed in the outpatient clinic area. It only took two or three months for Candy to improve enough to no longer need hospital care.

The clinic area where she was to receive the remainder of her therapy was huge. There were always many children in the waiting room on clinic days. Some of the children were receiving medications. Others were waiting their turn to be seen and still others were playing happily. Often, brothers and sisters of patients enthusiastically joined the activities. Usually one or two of the children were upset or crying either because they were afraid about what was about to happen or they still had pain from what had already been done.

The waiting area was always bustling, busy and noisy. Despite all the hubbub, Candy's screams could easily be heard above the roar created by the crowd assembled in the clinic almost from the moment she and her parents walked through the swinging doors at the front entrance.

Waiting to be seen was always an ordeal for her. Finally her name would be called and she would head with her family back to the hidden and dreaded treatment room. That treatment room must have seemed like a torture chamber. The treatment tables were long wooden frames with a padded cushion on top. Connected to the four corner support legs, a few feet off the floor, was a flat piece of wood that could serve as a storage shelf. Candy would use that shelf as a convenient place to hide. She would crawl onto the narrow piece of wood and grab tightly onto one of the two wooden legs closest to the wall. Talking, pleading, bribing and coercing only caused her to increase her grip and her crying. After about 10-15 minutes of trying to coax her out, two to three people would pull her out from underneath the table and position her on the padded cushion on top of the table.

Once she had been forcibly moved onto the treatment table, at least four strong adults would be needed to hold her down. She would be placed into a lying position on her side with her face looking at the wall. Her dress would be pulled up over her shoulders and her panties would be pulled down below her buttocks. The view that greeted me when I would enter the room was a bare back that almost convulsively moved in and out, up and down. Several adults would be holding the bucking back with red faces and sweat on their brows. I was expected to perform the necessary spinal tap under these seemingly barbaric conditions. I would work hard to move my hands in the same rhythm as her flailing back in order to clean her back in a sterile manner. If she or one of the holders had not managed to contaminate my sterile field, I would inject a local anesthetic into her back to numb the area where the spinal needle would soon go. The adrenaline surge brought on by her anxiety made it impossible for her to calm down. Her screams of terror were bone chilling and would cause my eardrums to ring.

Although four or five adults were holding, or, by this time, literally sitting on top of her, she continued to wiggle and jerk her back like a frightened bronco at a rodeo. Inserting the spinal needle was fraught with danger and difficulty. Matching the needle to the planned location while the area moved in all directions was sheer luck. Somehow, despite all the immense difficulty, the procedure would be completed. Once the spinal needle was removed, the adult holders would relax their grips just a bit. This would be the signal to the frightened child that she had made it through another dreaded spinal tap and she would begin to stop fighting just a bit. Her body would slowly relax probably more from fatigue than from relief. The sessions were always nerve-wracking and dreadful. I would be anxious for at least a week before whenever I saw that Candy was due for a spinal tap. After the procedure was finally over, I would be shaking and my shirt would be sweat-stained.

Shortly before I finished my training, Candy received her last spinal tap and stopped therapy. I vowed that once I went somewhere else to practice, I would not allow a child to suffer as I knew Candy had. I do not know what became of Candy. I believe that she was cured of her leukemia. Still, I wonder whether she ever recovered from the psychological assaults inflicted upon her in order to produce that cure. Somehow it does not make a lot of sense to me to *produce* pain and suffering in order to *relieve* pain and suffering.

Once I left my training to enter the Air Force, I began to look for a short-acting, effective sedative. I felt that children undergoing painful procedures would be best served if they were asleep during the time it took to perform those procedures. The medicine needed to last for only 5 to 10 minutes, needed to be safe and needed to have few side effects.

One of the pediatric cardiologists I worked with had been searching for the same sort of sedative so that he could study the hearts of his patients while the children slept. He suggested that I try *Ketamine*. He used it on his patients and found that it provided the type of pain relief that I was looking for. Ketamine is a very interesting medication that was originally developed as an anesthetic for use by veterinarians. It produces a *dissociative anesthesia*. This means that the person continues to breathe and retain control over their airway, but is unaware of painful events that are occurring. The medicine also produces amnesia for a period of time ranging from a few minutes to as long as a half-hour following its administration. With this medication the person does not remember undergoing painful procedures. In addition, the child will not stop breathing or choke on saliva like he or she might with other anesthetics. Each child reacts differently to the medication. Some stay under its effects for a long period or take a long time to recover from the sedation it produces. Some wake up in wonderful, almost euphoric moods, while others wake up in wild, almost uncontrollable states. There are two problems with this medication. The first is that it causes the child to increase saliva production. This can cause drooling or even choking. I do not allow the children to eat or drink anything for at least two hours before they receive the Ketamine. About one hour before they receive the sedative, they are given *atropine*. Atropine dries the mouth. This decreases the risk that the child will develop problems from the increased salivation.

The other problem with Ketamine is that some children experience hallucinations as they wake up. Sometimes the visions are pleasant and sometimes they have a nightmarish quality. Because hallucinations are more common in teenagers and adults, the medication is generally not recommended for older patients. Because of some of the bizarre reactions I witnessed when I first began using Ketamine, I searched for another sedative medication. I wanted a drug that would allow me to give the Ketamine at a lower dose but still give the child adequate sedation.

About twelve years ago I found that I could combine Ketamine with *Nembutol*, a short-acting barbiturate. This combination allowed me to decrease the doses of both medications without losing the benefit of either. I have found this combination of drugs to be very effective. In the years in which I have used this sedation combination, I have only had three patients who did not respond adequately. One child did not achieve sedation despite what I felt was a dose of medicines that was more than I was comfortable giving. A second child developed decreased oxygen levels shortly after the medicines were given. Even though he recovered his color quickly, the experience was one that I did not wish to repeat. A third child had a prolonged period of hallucinations and I felt that he should not receive Ketamine a second time. Each of these children subsequently received their procedures at an outpatient surgery center under the watchful eye of a trained anesthesiologist. These children still managed to get excellent pain relief but at a substantial cost increase as well as added inconvenience.

Some of the reactions that occur as the children awaken from the combination of the Ketamine and the Nembutol have been humorous. Willy was a 4-year old boy with ALL. He used to go to sleep prior to bone marrow studies or spinal taps with a great big smile on his face. Once when he woke up, he turned to me and began to sing, "You must have been a beautiful baby." I am sure that his parents must have sung that to him, but the sight of a somewhat drunk-behaving 4-year old singing that old-fashioned song was rather funny.

Some children and adolescents are old enough and mature enough to make their own decision as to whether they will have painful procedures performed while they are awake. I think that such young persons should be allowed to decide for themselves how they want to have invasive procedures performed. Some of my patients have decided that they do not want to be sedated for invasive procedures such as bone marrow studies or spinal taps. To these children, the loss of control induced by the sedation is worse than the potential pain of the procedure. The nurses and I provide lots of support to those who decide to have procedures done while awake. Since the children themselves have made the decision, they usually do very well without sedation.

One of the strangest effects of Ketamine is that most of the children go to sleep very rapidly and with their eyes open. If the parents or others in the room observing are not prepared, this can be quite unnerving. Kathy is a young lady who was diagnosed about eight years ago with ALL. The first few times she had a bone marrow examination or a spinal tap performed, the procedures were done in a treatment room or a surgical suite at the hospital. Kathy's mother had always stepped out of the room when the procedure was about to start. Ten days after starting chemotherapy, Kathy had improved to the point that she was able to go home.

A bone marrow study and a spinal tap were scheduled for the 14th day of therapy. Kathy was frightened since this was the first time she had been in the office. She wanted her mother to stay with her until she fell asleep. Kathy's mother wanted to be anywhere but in that room, but she very gamely stayed at her daughter's side. The little girl's central venous catheter was easily accessed and a dose of Nembutol was slowly given. Kathy became somewhat dizzy and tired and she lay down on the treatment table. My nurse then slowly pushed a dose of Ketamine. Within about 20 seconds after the medication had been flushed into her bloodstream, the little girl's eyelids began to flutter and her eyes opened wide. She did not respond to us, but she was in no distress. Her respiratory pattern remained smooth and clear and her skin color remained pink. Her mother, however, was not doing quite as well. She took one look at the sedated child, turned white and ran screaming from the room. I did not have time to find out what had happened since Ketamine is very short acting and there were two painful procedures to be done. Swiftly and expertly the bone marrow aspiration and the spinal tap were finished and Kathy was carried into a nearby bedroom to recover from the effects of the medications. I sat with the child while Marian went to find her mother. Marian found her in a corner of the lady's room, clutching an unlit cigarette, crying and shaking. Marian brought her back to sit at her sleeping daughter's bedside. After we finally convinced Kathy's anxious mother that her daughter was fine, she told us why she had reacted as she did. The prior evening she had experienced a nightmare in which her daughter had died. When the dream funeral was held, the little girl's eyes had been open. The Ketamine had caused Kathy to become unresponsive. Despite being asleep and sedated, her eyes were wide open. When her mother saw her in that state, she was convinced that her nightmare had come true. Seeing that Kathy was fine and beginning to awaken relieved her of her fear. Since that time, we have been careful to warn the parents what to expect so as not to experience such a reaction again.

Kathy turned out to be a child who would awaken rapidly after receiving Ketamine. As soon as she was even somewhat alert, she was ready to leave. Unfortunately, she was only ready to go in her own mind. Even though she was still under the influence of the medication and quite dizzy and unsteady, she would get out of the bed and try to walk. At times it was a bit funny since she would look like a drunk driver failing a sobriety test. However, I was always concerned that she would walk into a wall or door in her somewhat inebriated state. Fortunately, she has been off all chemotherapy for more than six years and is now cured of leukemia. She no longer needs sedation.

Ketamine is not the only medication that can be used to sedate children for invasive or painful procedures. There are several that have been and are being used by children's cancer programs all around the world. Regardless of which medications are used, some method must be available to protect the children from pain and anxiety. When I was in medical school, we used to say that a doctor who did procedures without any sedation was using the anesthetics, *Okaine* or *Brutaine*. Okaine worked like this. The child was held down so that he or she could not move. The doctor, nurse or other support personnel would say over and over, "It's okay! Just hang on! It's okay! It will be over soon, okay? It's okay!"

Those words might have made the doctor or nurse feel better, but they did little for the child. Brutaine was identical to Okaine except no comments were made. Brutaine meant that the procedure was done in the same way it would be if the child were being mauled by a brute. Such pseudo-pain control methods are really a form of assault. As an advocate for children, I cannot participate in such child abuse. Some parents want to be present when their children have a painful test done. Others would just as soon not witness the procedure. Some children act more anxious when their parents are not in the room while others are calmed by the presence of their mother or father. I leave the decision whether the parents remain in the treatment room up to the child and the parents. I know that I feel better when I can witness what is happening to my own children. I think the practice of insisting that parents leave when the child is undergoing a painful examination can be more stressful for the child or for the parents and may lead to resentment and anger.

One of the myths of pain control is that the doctor needs to be very concerned that the child might become a drug addict. Certainly no one who lives in America could be unaware of the drug problem that currently exists among our nation's youth. Still, it is very unusual for a pediatrician or pediatric oncologist to have to deal with a patient who has become a drug addict as a result of having received pain medication. Most of the children do not like feeling out of control and that is exactly how medications like Morphine, Demerol, Ketamine and Nembutol make them feel. As soon as their pain is gone, most children are happy to stop taking the pain medications. There is little reason not to do everything possible to provide adequate pain relief. Procedures are one of the important things that can produce pain, but tumors and disease progression can also result in severe pain. There are so many ways that have been developed to provide pain relief that it is rare that someone should have to be in pain even in the terminal phases of a cancer.

I strongly disagree with those who believe that doctors should be allowed to assist terminal patients to commit suicide. Providing adequate pain control is often frustrating, rarely lucrative and usually time-consuming. Many doctors are not terribly interested in this aspect of care and so there are many patients who have received and still do receive inadequate support for painful conditions. Recognition of this problem is growing and the problem of adequate pain control is now being addressed in many cancer centers. Still, much more work needs to be done to ensure that children with cancer do not suffer from needless pain.

I believe that the correct amount of pain medication is whatever dose is needed to relieve the patient's pain. David taught me that lesson quite vividly. When David was found to have a tumor growing in the back of his right eye, his parents took him to an eye expert in Philadelphia. The tumor, a retinoblastoma, was a rare malignancy found almost always in young children. This tumor is important to oncologists because it has enabled cancer experts to learn a great deal about the genetics of cancer. The cure rate for this tumor is high if it is caught early. The ophthalmologist in Philadelphia who examined David felt that he would have the best chance to be cured if the eye with the cancerous tumor was removed and replaced with a prosthesis. Other pediatric doctors in Philadelphia reviewed David's case and decided that he did not need to have any other therapy at that time.

Five months after his eye was removed, David developed a painful lump on his forehead just above his right eyebrow. The surgeon in his hometown performed a biopsy of the lump. The pathology examination showed that the retinoblastoma had recurred and had spread from the boy's eye into his skull bones. Within a short time, three more lumps suddenly appeared on the little boy's head. David was sent to me to see what could be done. When I first met him and his family, they were frightened. I tried to reassure them the best that I could. After a brief visit and examination in my office, I admitted the handsome towheaded little boy to the hospital so that further studies could be done. Those examinations showed that retinoblastoma cells were growing in several sites in his body. I found cancer cells in several of his bones as well as more cells hiding in his bone marrow. Chemotherapy offered the best hope for delaying or even stopping the rapid and aggressive growth of the malignancy. Despite my usual optimistic outlook, I knew that history was against us. While responses had been reported in children with retinoblastomas that had spread from the eye, the number of children who had been cured once the tumor had spread was very small. Still, David, his parents, his sisters and I embarked on therapy on the hope that David would be the one to beat the devastatingly poor odds.

David's response to the first course of intensive chemotherapy medications was dramatic. The lumps on his forehead seemed to practically melt away and he began to feel better. David was from a small town where cattle ranching, hunting and fishing were the way of life. He was a true cowboy. Marian quickly fell in love with him. He remained very quiet and scared around me for a long time. I think he had the idea that I might try to snatch his only good eye when he was not paying attention. David would spend many hours talking about riding horses, roping and branding cattle with Marian and she would listen with enthusiasm. He always laughed at tier because she was such a city slicker and did not understand his world. I knew that chemotherapy and even radiation to the obvious areas of involvement were unlikely to cure this cute little boy. I recommended to his family that we pursue the option of a bone marrow transplant. David's parents were not sure that they wanted their son to undergo such an intensive and dangerous treatment even if it were the only way for him to be cured. It did not matter anyway. His insurance company declared that the procedure was experimental and refused to pay for it. When I told them about the insurance company's decision, they were actually relieved that the decision had been taken out of their hands. Every four weeks David would come to the office to get a chemotherapy treatment. Despite the intensity of the medicines and all of the potential side effects, he continued to be free of pain. His forehead remained flat and his bone marrow became clear of the dreaded cells. He was able to play and join his father in his work with the cows and goats and horses on the ranch. David entered kindergarten six months after chemotherapy was instituted.

The same week that he was supposed to start school he was due to begin a new course of therapy. Her mother did not want anything to interfere with his kindergarten experience and requested that his schedule be altered. As a result, the chemotherapy was delayed for one week to allow him to enjoy his first week of school. David enjoyed school almost as much as working the cattle with his father. About 15 months after he had first appeared in my office came the day that I most feared. In the time that I had known him, David had changed from a scared, scrawny little boy with funny bumps on his forehead to a bright, confident and happy young man. The phone call I received one Thursday morning from the boy's mother told me that all the good we had achieved in the previous 15 months was about to end. She told me that David was complaining of some pain while chewing. This did not bother me so much right then as there were several reasons why he might complain of such a problem. Then she added that he was also having nightmares and waking up in the middle of the night screaming in terror. When he had first developed the lumps on his forehead, he had initially complained of nightmares. I knew that his symptoms scared his mother for she feared (as did I) that the tumor had returned. I made a space in my schedule to see him the next morning.

The X-rays of his chin were disappointing and disheartening. On one of the X-ray views, a small defect could be seen in the bone of the lower jaw. X-rays taken just three months earlier had not shown any such change. I tried to maintain some optimism. There might be another explanation for the X-ray defect but a biopsy soon confirmed that retinoblastoma cells were again growing in David's jawbone. The retinoblastoma had only toyed with us. The tumor cells had responded long enough to get our hopes up. Seeing the abnormal X-ray and then reading the biopsy report felt like falling off a mountain peak with no supporting rope to protect us on the way down. Shortly after the results of the biopsy reached me, I sat down with the child's parents and reviewed the options. Already they had decided privately what they would do if the tumor ever recurred. They had experienced enough of chemotherapy and treatments. They desired nothing more than that David could be made as comfortable and pain-free for as long as possible. David thought that not having to receive any more chemotherapy was pretty nifty. He returned to kindergarten as if nothing had changed. In fact, nothing had really changed for him other than he was no longer having to travel to my office every 4 weeks and was no longer getting sick from the chemotherapy. A few weeks passed with no problems but then his jaw began to ache a bit more. Radiation was given to the jaw area where his pain was the worst. The radiation was not designed to cure the tumor because the retinoblastoma cells were actively growing again in all parts of his bone marrow. The radiation could only treat the one small part of the little boy's body where his pain was most intense. Radiation used under such circumstances can often provide excellent palliation. The tumor remained fairly stable for the remainder of the school year. David missed only a few days of kindergarten.

Kindergarten graduation day was a special day mixed with many ambiguous feelings for David's parents. They were so proud of their son as he crossed the room to have his special achievement acknowledged, but they also were enormously sad because they knew that this graduation would be the only one in which he would ever participate David was the youngest child in a family of proud and independent people. Before David became sick they had found little reason to ask or depend on others for help or support. Their resolve and strength came from within. Once David's tumor grew back, Marian suggested that the child might enjoy a wish from the Make-A-Wish organization. David's mother would say that she liked the idea of going on vacation, but she would make all sorts of excuses to keep from making the trip. She was a schoolteacher and tried to schedule the trip once school let out for the summer. Marian kept trying to let her know that David might not be in any condition to wait until summer. David's wish was for a trip to the mountains.

Finally, the family got everything together and prepared for their trip. David's only concern was that he might see some bears and bears scared him. The trip was a special tonic for the anxiety and pressure with which the family had been constantly living. For several days they had fun as a family without having to think about cancer, treatments or death. David was at just the right place when they left. He was well enough so that he enjoyed the vacation immensely. For a short time, fear and pain were not a part of his life. His week in the mountains passed all too quickly. Fortunately, no bears showed up to disturb the peaceful nature of their journey. The tumor, however, was not deterred by the trip and even seemed to be stimulated by the mountain air. Right around the time that the family returned, his right arm began to ache and a new growth was found near his elbow. Soon after he again began to complain about his lower jaw. In a short period, it became clear that the tumor was also growing again there. Pain management now became much more important.

Many new agents and ways of giving pain medications have been developed over the past several years. The problem in the management of pain comes in trying to work out which single agent or combinations of medications will provide the best relief for each individual. It is also difficult to oversee pain management and respond to new episodes of pain over the telephone or from long distances away. David's family wanted him to stay at home. The hospital experiences had been traumatic for him and his family. David was afraid of hospitals. Other than Marian, he did not trust any of the nurses. He knew that in the hospital people did things that hurt him or made him sick. At home he could go with his father to help care for the farm animals or sit and play with his mother and sisters. David's sisters were both teenagers. The older of the two tried to separate herself from the illness and death which now pervaded the house. This created many conflicts within the family.

Such conflicts are normal for any home with a teenager, but David's illness magnified and focused her normal teenage tendencies. David's younger sister, on the other hand, waited on her brother as if she was his private duty nurse. She put aside all of her needs to take care of his. The two sisters would not have been as easily understood or accommodated in a hospital setting. Since the family lived so far from where I had my practice, it was difficult to provide the kind of support they needed. I had called a hospice program headquartered in their hometown, but the family never hit it off with the hospice nurses. Under such intimate and painful circumstances, a close bond must be established between the patient, the family and the hospice personnel. David, however, did not like the hospice nurses. They were more used to working with adults and the special needs of children scared them. David was already afraid of nurses anyway and he could sense their tentativeness. He would go further into his shell whenever the hospice nurses came by for a visit. David's mother was already providing pretty much all of his medical care. Within a few weeks, she asked that the nurses stop coming by. I believe that the hospice nurses were as relieved by that request as the family was.

Even without nurses, the little boy still needed IV's and medications. These were provided by a home health care agency. Once a week the home heath care delivery truck would drive up the long dirt driveway that led to the family home and drop off the necessary supplies. We would call from the office to give advice and support. Initially we only spoke a few times a week. But as the tumor began to grow and cause more pain, we communicated more often. Pain control began with *acetaminophen* and *ibuprofen* products. These quickly became inadequate and stronger medicines were soon added.

The first attempt to control the increasing pain was a *narcotic patch*. These patches are fairly new devices. They look something like small plastic bandages. The medicine contained in the bandage is absorbed slowly and continuously over a two to three day period. The patches are nice since they only need to be changed every two to three days and no medicine needs to be injected or swallowed. The other advantage is that they supply a continuous small amount of pain medicine so that the person always has some pain medication in their system.

The patches have the same disadvantages inherent in all narcotic analgesics. People on narcotics often complain of itching, constipation, and sleepiness. There are many other potential and real side effects that these people may have. Sometimes the side effects are bad enough that they seem to be worse than the pain itself. This is quite unusual. Narcotics are usually very effective at controlling pain but they are not without their downside. The patches have an additional potential negative. They can irritate the skin since they stay in the same place for several days. The patches worked well for David. He did not like to take medicine by mouth since that hurt his already sore and swollen jaw and usually he would object to the taste. His parents did not want to bother with his catheter because they were afraid that a needle and dressing in his chest and a chronically running IV might interfere with his ability to participate in those activities he enjoyed and still felt up to doing.

A few months after returning from their trip to the mountains, while he still felt fairly well, a local stock show and rodeo was held in David's hometown. Each year the children of the area would raise a farm animal to exhibit for competition. After the judging was completed, the animals would be auctioned off. It was a way for the children to learn how to raise farm animals and for them to make a little money while doing so. David had been raising a lamb he had named Pudge. He had been unable to give Pudge much attention because the lamb required more time than a sick, little boy could provide. A few days before Pudge was to be judged, a friend of David's family phoned Marian. She explained that the lamb was not in very good shape. She was afraid that the lamb would not be bid on at the auction and thought that such an outcome might hurt David's feelings. Even though Pudge had been somewhat neglected, he was still David's pride and joy. Marian and I agreed that we would offer up to $300.00 for Pudge as long as no one else made a bid. A few days later we were the reluctant owners of a somewhat bedraggled lamb. Ours was the only bid for Pudge. Since the only thing we knew about lambs was that Mary had once owned one, we donated Pudge to David and his family. It had cost us $300.00, but it was worth it. We had made a little boy very happy.

Eventually David's pain worsened and even the patches were not enough. *Morphine* was then added to the mix of medications. First it was given under his tongue from where it could be absorbed into his bloodstream. This worked fairly well for a while, but David objected to the medicine's bitter taste. He had to be in terrible pain before he would agree to take it. Having run out of simple alternatives, it became clear that intravenous narcotics were now needed to control the child's advancing pain. Just as we were about to start him on occasional *boluses* of intravenous morphine, the family received an unexpected offer for a trip similar to the Make A Wish trip to the mountains. Special events and visits with admired people have a way of reducing pain and anxiety so that one may enjoy him or herself without the pain ruining the good time. Once the episode is over, exhaustion and pain usually return full force.

One particularly gray day late in the summer, the family received a phone call from the publicist for a major film star. A friend of the family had written to the star about David. This actor had played David's favorite character in a very successful made-for-television movie. David would watch the movie over and over on videotape. That actor was David's ultimate hero. David's story had touched the actor who was usually very private and reserved. He had heard about the child while in the hills of Wyoming filming the sequel to the original movie. He invited David and his family to join him for a weekend while the movie was being made. David's mother called me before agreeing to go. She wanted to know if it would be safe for David to travel that far. I told her that if they did not go, I would. With that ringing endorsement of the trip, the family left the next day for the remote location to meet this famous star. David required virtually no pain medications during the entire weekend. It is amazing what good pain relievers such trips can be. All of the adrenaline and excitement of the trip wore off within a few hours of the family's return to reality. It did not take long before David was again suffering from the full brunt of the pain.

In the final few weeks of his life, David only rarely was able to go out to enjoy his favorite activities. At the time, my nephew Craig was working at a shooting range. He knew David and knew that David enjoyed hunting. The problem was that a full-sized rifle was too big and strong for a little boy, especially one with a sore jaw and arm. Craig borrowed a cut-down rifle from the child of one of his friends and gave it to David to use. David loved the rifle. The day after Craig delivered his special gift, David, his father and Craig went hunting together. Once again the excitement and distraction of something special was quite effective at pain relief. The next day, however. David was too exhausted even to get out of bed. Every night after that he slept with the rifle but only used it that one time. That rifle, just like the visit to the movie star and the bear-less visit to the mountains served as a great pain reliever.

The last few weeks of David's life were less exciting. Marian drove the three hours to his house to see her little cowboy about 14 days before his death. Seeing Marian was very special for David, but it was very hard on Marian. Her little cowboy had changed drastically. His jaw was now swollen to almost unrecognizable proportions. He was in obvious pain and it broke her heart to see him in that condition. Marian knew that the time had come for David to receive the Morphine on a regular basis through his intravenous catheter. Within a few hours of her visit, the intravenous medicine was started. David's parents were given permission to increase the dose of the morphine whenever they felt that David needed more medicine in order to remain comfortable. Every day, and sometimes twice or even three times a day, we would talk to David's family to provide support. Marian did most of the communicating. At first David's mother was reluctant to increase the morphine. She would call each time her son's pain seemed to increase and ask what she should do. I finally convinced her that there was no maximum dose as long as David was still in pain. Initially only 1 mg. of morphine per hour was adequate to provide relief. By the time he died, the Morphine was running at 200 mg. per hour. Even at that very high dose he was awake and able to let his parents know that he was comfortable. He could not move his mouth or his right arm because of the tumor, but he was not in pain. The ability to control the pain and the pain medications at home gave David's parents a great deal of comfort. They knew that no one could have provided as much love and support to their child as they had. David's death was both a great sadness and a relief.

His parents had watched his torment and knew that his suffering was finally at an end. Even though we were not able to be with the family at the time of David's death nor join them at the funeral, I feel that Marian, Craig and I made a big difference in David's life. We have no control to stop a tumor from growing nor can we ensure that the tumor will go away permanently, but we do have the control to make life a little bit better for a sick child and for his or her family. We not only have the control; we have the obligation to do so.

Pain management in the home is a relatively new and somewhat controversial area. Most lay people (and actually many doctors and nurses) feel that people who take narcotics such as morphine have a high risk of becoming addicted. True addiction is actually quite rare. It is reported to occur in no more than 1% of patients on chronic narcotic therapy. It is important to distinguish between *tolerance* and *dependence*. People on morphine for a few days will begin to develop tolerance. This means that they will begin to require higher doses to achieve the same degree of pain relief. They also may develop withdrawal symptoms when the medication is removed. Neither the need for higher doses over a prolonged time period to achieve the same effect nor withdrawal symptoms are signs of drug dependence. Drug dependence means that the person has developed active drug-seeking behaviors. Most people on narcotics take them because that is the only way that their pain symptoms can be relieved. I have found that the vast majority of children hate the way the narcotics make them feel. They do not like the feelings of nausea, itching, lethargy and sleepiness that accompany the use of morphine. Once the pain is gone, they have few problems physically or emotionally with eliminating the narcotics from their regimens.

Having the parents manage the intravenous narcotics at home raises some further problems. The first issue is to ensure that the medicine gets from the pharmacy that mixes it to the home where it is to be used. If the child lives in a neighborhood where drugs are commonly abused, the person who delivers the narcotics could become an easy target for robbery if it becomes known what he or she is delivering. It is recommended that the delivery be made in unmarked vehicles rather than advertising the name of the pharmacy on the car or truck. What should the doctor do if one of the parents or a family member is a drug abuser? How does that physician ensure that the narcotics actually get delivered to the child? I have actually had to deal with this exact situation.

Many years ago while I was serving my time in the Air Force, I took care of a sweet 7-year old named Courtney. Courtney had developed severe pain in her right hip and had been taken by her mother and stepfather to see their local Air Force doctor. At the time they had been living on a remote base. The doctor examined the child and obtained a plain X-ray of the hip. The hipbone on the right side was nearly completely eaten away by an aggressive and nasty cancer known as a neuroblastoma. The bone looked like a sweater that had been devoured by a band of hungry moths.

Neuroblastoma is a cancer of the sympathetic nervous system. It occurs in young children and often is widely spread when found. Although treatments and outcomes have improved since my days with the Air Force, it still is a very difficult cancer for pediatric oncologists. At the time that Courtney was diagnosed, only about 5% of the children with metastatic neuroblastoma could be expected to be disease-free at least two years from diagnosis. Within 24 hours after the doctor took a look at that original X-ray, Courtney and her family were transferred to my base so that she could receive appropriate care. The neuroblastoma had started in the little girl's right adrenal gland and had spread wildly from there into many of her bones and bone marrow. Courtney had a very large amount of cells growing rapidly in her body and a very bad prognosis. Within a few days of her arrival, Courtney was started on chemotherapy. Like most children with neuroblastoma, she initially had a good response. Her pains improved and her personality and behavior returned to normal. About seven months passed as her condition continued to improve.

Then, one day without warning, she began to limp. Two days later the pain in her hip was as bad as it had been originally. The neuroblastoma had recurred. This time it was even nastier and more aggressive. Courtney's parents were at first interested in exploring new experimental treatments. They tried one but when it only made the child feel horrible and did nothing to stop the growth of the aggressive cancer, they opted to take their child home in hospice care. Pain is a major problem for children with progressive neuroblastoma. The ability to have such children at home relatively free of suffering usually depends on the adequacy of pain control. Courtney's parents were very willing to help their child. They were realistic. They knew that their beloved and beautiful child was going to die and they wanted her to die at home.

There was one major problem. Courtney's aunt (her mother's sister) was a heroin addict. I spoke at length with Courtney's mother and with the pharmacist about the ethical, legal and medical questions that would arise as a result of keeping large amounts of morphine in the family home. Together we made plans how best to monitor the medicine. I then had a conversation with Courtney's aunt. She was well aware of the potential problems her addiction caused for her niece. I made it clear that if she did anything with the morphine that was there for Courtney's use that she would not be given a second chance. She promised to abide by our rules. I spent many hours in Courtney's home during the last several weeks of her life. She was kept at a good comfort level by her parent's diligent care. Despite her aunt's history, the morphine syringe count was never off. Courtney died peacefully on a Friday morning. Her parents were as prepared as possible when the child left this mortal life. When I arrived at the home, there was a sense of calm and peace. Shortly after I pronounced the child and made sure the family members were okay, Courtney's drug-addicted aunt gathered up the remaining unused vials of morphine and handed them to me. The count matched. Not a single vial was missing. When I left the home later that afternoon, I took the morphine with me back to the Air Force Base to discard it. I was very pleased with what had happened with Courtney's aunt. Later she told me that her experience with her niece was the most profound and important of her life. She used her newfound strength to kick her habit and has remained clean since. Unfortunately, her story is an exception.

Pain control can work well when the parents are cooperative and only desire relief for their child. Vanessa, however, taught me that not all parents were as wonderful as David's or Courtney's. Vanessa was 15 years old when she was diagnosed with a very rare malignant ovarian tumor. She had initially started her therapy at a cancer center in another city. The doctors there had determined that intensive chemotherapy following surgery would be the best way to prevent the tumor from recurring. Vanessa's white blood cell count would drop significantly a week or two after she received each treatment. In order to try and keep her from developing severe infections when her white blood cell count was at its nadir, the doctors at the cancer center used a new medicine known as GCSF to help her bone marrow recover quicker.

GCSF had been released for use in the United States right around the time that Vanessa had been diagnosed. GCSF does not change the chemotherapy's effect on bone marrow production of white blood cells. It works by enhancing the rate at which the bone marrow makes new white blood cells. One of the side effects of GCSF is that it can produce bone pain in some patients. For most people the bone pain can be managed with mild analgesics such as ibuprofen or acetaminophen. Rarely, some patients require stronger pain medications to control the pain. Vanessa seemed to be such a person. Because of the severity of the pain she reported, Vanessa had narcotic analgesics prescribed.

A few months after she started therapy, Vanessa and her family moved to a city nearer to my office. Her father called to ask if his daughter could continue her treatment in my office. Vanessa was a lovely young lady. She wore a long, curly, blonde wig to hide her baldness. The wig made her look like a country-western singing star. She was articulate and funny but she had a fairly cynical attitude toward life. I was sometimes shocked by her adult view of the world along with her "street smarts." I have always been somewhat naive about other's motives. I practically have to be hit by a truck to believe that someone could be deliberately deceptive or dishonest. In this day and age, I am not sure that my innocent outlook on life is totally healthy, but it has served me well to this point. Vanessa was in some ways my alter-ego. She was as non-trusting and non-believing as I was naive and gullible. In her worldliness I found her to be very interesting. Despite the fact that she always appeared happy whenever she came to my office, her parents continued to tell me that her bone pain was severe. They continued to insist that she needed pain relief. I continued to supply the medication they said she needed because I believed them. They seemed very concerned that their daughter's pain was continuing as severely as it was. Pain is very subjective. I usually have very little reason not to believe someone when they say they are in pain. About 3 months after I started caring for her, a pharmacist from her hometown expressed his concern to me about the large amount of pain relievers that Vanessa was requiring. I explained to him about her problem, but I must admit that I was also becoming more suspicious.

The next time her father called to renew the prescription, I asked him whether he was concerned that Vanessa was continuing to need so much medicine. Instead of reacting with concern, as I expected, he became angry that I would even suggest that there might be a problem with overuse or abuse of medication. This definitely raised my suspicions even more. I began to think that the problem was with Vanessa's father and not with her. I figured that he might be using or selling the pain medicine, but I had no proof and no way to verify my feelings. About two weeks later, the proof arrived. I was working in my office one afternoon trying to dig out from under a huge pile of overdue reports and letters. A person called but refused to give her name. My office staff knows that I like to make my own decision as to whether I will take a phone call directly or take a message and call back later. The woman had said only that she had some information that I would find important. I had a free moment and so I had my receptionist put her through. The anonymous woman told me that she had a neighbor whose daughter was being treated for cancer and that I was the child's doctor. She went on to add that she knew that the parents were asking for and receiving prescriptions for powerful pain relievers but that the child was not taking them. She would not give me the child's name, but I knew that she could only be talking about one family. I was very disappointed that my suspicions had proven to be true. I thanked her for the information. Before she hung up she made me promise that I would not disclose the source of my information.

The next day Vanessa and her parents came to the hospital since it was time for her to start the next cycle of chemotherapy. When I arrived at the nursing station, I recruited two nurses and a social worker to accompany me into her room. I wanted to make sure there were several witnesses to the discussion that was about to occur. I was nervous. I had never confronted a family about such a problem before. Vanessa was already lying down on the bed on top of the covers. The head of the bed was elevated. Long, curly blond hair from Vanessa's wig cascaded over the raised pillow. I told her hello and asked her family to sit down in chairs placed at the side of the bed. I sat down on the edge of the bed where I could look directly into Vanessa's and her parent's eyes. I took a deep breath. My hands were shaking and my heart was pounding as I told the family that I knew that Vanessa was not using the pain medications that I had been prescribing. I paused a moment and then asked her parents which of them were using the drugs. Both of the parents immediately became defensive and angry. They looked me straight in the face as they said that they could not believe that I would accuse them of such behavior. I replied that I not only believed that they were using the drugs, but that I knew that it was happening. They continued to deny that they would ever do anything to hurt their child, but I remained adamant. I finally told them about the phone calls I had received. I explained to them my suspicions had been aroused by the first call from their pharmacist. I did not tell them the source for the second call, but they guessed anyway. I did not confirm whether they had guessed correctly, but their reaction was to become angry with their neighbor. I thought it odd that the major target for their anger was the person who had told on them.

After several tense and angry minutes, Vanessa's mother finally admitted that they had not given the pain medications to their daughter. Even after her mother's admission, I was fascinated that Vanessa continued to insist that she was taking the medication. It must have been an extremely difficult situation for the teenager. She not only had to deal with the fact that her parents were abusing drugs, but now she had to deal with the fact that other people were well aware of their problem. Perhaps the only way for her to cope with the very volatile situation was to continue to claim that her mother was lying and she had been taking the medicines as prescribed. Despite her protests, the pretense was over. I had thought that Vanessa's father was the one who had the drug problem, but it turned out that both of her parents were using me to supply their habits. I tried to be non-judgmental although I was angry that I had been used in such a way. I told them that I could no longer give their child prescriptions that would be misused. I said that I was willing to help them find treatment if they desired such support. I was very clear with them that Vanessa truly did have a serious cancer and continued to need therapy.

After admitting that they both had a serious problem, both mother and father told me that they could not go for drug rehabilitation without losing their jobs. They expressed no real desire to change. Like most drug abusers, they took little responsibility for their own actions. The confrontation had gone just as I had hoped it would. Now we were at a point where the parents needed to decide if they wanted to get help for their serious problem. They asked for some time alone with their daughter so they could discuss what they should do. The nurses and the social worker were in a state of shock. I had not informed them prior to this confrontation what to expect. I do not believe that they had any idea that such a problem existed. I think that they, like myself, had difficulty believing that any parent would use their child's illness as a pretext to get drugs. Within a few minutes of the parent's request for some private time, we all went out to the nursing desk to wait. I was somewhat shaky but glad that I had confronted the situation. While we were at the nursing station quietly discussing how we should proceed, the family came out of the room. Without saying a word to anyone, they quickly left the floor. I was not totally surprised by this move, but the others sitting there were shocked. No one made a move to stop them. None of us really knew what to do.

The next morning I called the doctor at the cancer center where Vanessa had been diagnosed and started therapy. I told her what had happened. She relayed to me that they had felt the same suspicions there but had not confronted the family because they lacked proof of drug abuse. The doctor felt that the family had left the cancer center not because they had moved but because the doctors there were about to stop prescribing the pain medication so freely. What made the situation so difficult was that Vanessa truly did have a rare and highly malignant cancer and she did need to receive treatment. Neither Vanessa nor her parents ever contacted me following the confrontation. They also did not return for cancer treatment at the original program. Five months after this event, I received a phone call from a doctor in a city about 4 hours away. He asked me what I knew about Vanessa. He told me that she had appeared at his office earlier that day. The history given by her parents was sadly familiar. Although she looked like she felt well and had a normal physical examination, her parents said that she was in excruciating pain. His instincts told him that something was not correct and he had called me to find out what was happening. I was very glad to hear that Vanessa was still well but very sad that her parents were continuing to use her cancer to support their own drug habits.

In spite of this very sad incident, I continue to believe that one of my major purposes as a pediatric oncologist is to relieve the pain and suffering of children as best I can. I hope I never again have to confront parents who would use their child's illness to satisfy their own needs.

Private Signals

Children are amazing. They are honest, forgiving, eager to give and receive love, fun, insightful, energetic and impulsive. Almost two out of every three children diagnosed with cancer this year will be cured (which is something no adult oncologist can say about his or her patients). It is the children that make this field such a special one.

I must admit that dealing with the families can sometimes be difficult. Perhaps thirty years ago, when families still resembled the Cleavers on "Leave It To Beaver" or the Stones on "The Donna Reed Show," it was easier. Now, such families are the exception. Mixed families, single parents, and divorce before, during and after the cancer has been diagnosed are the norm. Since I grew up in a traditional family (mother and father together) and I currently live in one, I have some trouble following some of the family relationships.

I recall one family where the mixing and matching of parents and children created some treatment difficulties. Amber was the youngest of seven children. She was being treated for ALL. Because of her condition, a bone marrow transplant represented the treatment of choice. The best chance for a successful transplant would be if one of her brothers or sisters were a match. I was encouraged that Amber had so many potential donors as that raised the chances that one of her six siblings would be a match for her. That was when I found out that things would not be so easy. After explaining the details about the matching process, I told Amber's parents that they needed to bring all of their children to the laboratory to have the blood tests drawn to see if any of the children matched Amber.

"That will be a bit of a problem," explained Amber's father. "My oldest son no longer lives at home."

"Can you reach him?" I asked.

"No," he answered. "His mother and I do not have a speaking relationship and I am not allowed to call my son."

"That's a shame," I replied, "but it probably is not necessary since it is obvious that your son has a different mother than Amber does. It is unlikely he would match her since he is only a half-brother."

"Is that important?" asked Amber's mother.

"Yes," I answered, "It's unlikely that a half-brother or half-sister would match."

"Well, then, we have a definite problem. I am the father of two of Amber's brothers and one of her sisters, but she is not their mother," said Amber's father pointing at Amber's mother.

"We not only have a problem with those three, but with the other three girls as well. They are my children, but they are not his," said Amber's mother pointing at Amber's father.

"Are there any children other than Amber that have both of you as parents?" I asked.

"Sorry to say, it appears that Amber is an only child," her father regretfully answered. We still tested most of Amber's half-brothers and half-sisters but none of them matched. The studies even suggested that her father had less of a biological relationship with the little girl than he thought, but discretion forced me not to discuss that situation further. This family is unfortunately not unique. A social worker is frequently required to help unravel some of these very complicated family relationships.

Determining parentage is not just a minor issue since a detailed and accurate family history may show such information as cancer risk in the child or even in other family members. Not only are the family genetics often very interesting and informative, but the relationships between family members are sometimes even more so. Some marriages are already headed for divorce even before the child is diagnosed with a serious or life-threatening illness. No matter how much energy or time we put into helping a family cope with the cancer diagnosis, we are unable to make such a family whole again. A bad relationship is only going to be made worse by the stress created by having to deal with the cancer.

Such was the case for Francine's family. Francine was 3 years old when she was diagnosed with ALL. I met the pretty child and her mother and father in the hospital one beautiful spring day. For a few days Francine's mother had been noticing that her daughter was bruising more than she thought was appropriate. After a few days of trying to rationalize the large number of bruises on her child's body, she had taken her to a pediatrician. The pediatrician had not only noticed the unusual purple spots but that the child was very pale. The pediatrician had ordered a blood count and was not totally surprised when the results suggested that the little girl had leukemia. He admitted the child to the hospital and called me to see her. When I entered the child's hospital room that afternoon, I was pleased to see both of her parents sitting at her bedside.

During the first few days of Francine's hospitalization, I discussed issues relating to leukemia and Francine's planned treatment. Her parents seemed very involved and caring, and I enjoyed working with them. Francine's father had short blond hair and the type of muscular body that comes only from performing physical labor. Although a man who had never attended college, he had the ability to understand the often complicated information that I was teaching him. His questions were always intelligent and well-reasoned. Her mother was a petite woman with attractive features. She was employed in a bank and had a mind which easily grasped the statistical information I presented. After spending several hours answering their questions and reviewing the plans, I felt that I knew both parents well.

The day before I had planned for Francine to go home, Marian came to her hospital room to meet the pretty little girl and talk with her parents. This was a way for her to establish a link between the hospital and the outpatient setting where she would receive most of the planned therapy. Her mother remained at her daughter's bedside. Her father had been required to return to work just the day before. Francine's mother arranged for a leave of absence from her work in order to remain with her daughter. She was almost enjoying the time away from the stressful business world. After introducing herself, Marian sat down with Francine's mother and talked about issues that might impact on the child's care. I had told Marian that Francine's father was a nice guy who had seemed very attentive toward his daughter and her older brother.

"I guess it's good that you have such a nice husband that you can rely on," Marian opened, trying gently to inquire about their relationship.

"That jerk!" Francine's mother spit back, "I couldn't rely on him if my life depended on it!"

Marian did not need any further information to realize that this was a relationship that was in deep trouble. The rift between the two parents, which was now evident, became much wider in the next few weeks. Despite my impressions that they were truly supportive of each other and of their children, Francine's mother and father had been having marital difficulties for months. Her father thought his wife was a demanding, controlling, hypercritical woman and she thought he was lazy, undependable and a very poor communicator. Their anger at each other had actually delayed their recognition of the slow but steady changes in their daughter that had finally resulted in her diagnosis of ALL. A few weeks after Francine's leukemia was discovered, her father moved out of the home into a nearby apartment. The two warring parents obtained a divorce just a few months later. I wish I could say that it was the end of the difficulties, but problems still remained.

Francine responded very well to the chemotherapy. One month after she started the medicines, she achieved a remission. Soon her condition had advanced to the point that she was able to return to the same activities that she had enjoyed before the leukemia had been found. Once her father moved out and even before the divorce decree was issued, Francine would sometimes stay with her father and sometimes with her mother. Francine seemed relatively unaffected by the change in her parent's situation, but her care was definitely affected. I did not care who came in with her since I liked both parents. The problem was that the communication between the two of them was so poor that it was nearly impossible to tell if the child's medications had been given correctly. Sometimes, one parent forgot to tell the other one about an appointment. When that happened, our receptionist would have to make several phone calls to find the parent who had the responsibility for Francine's care for that day. After a while, we got a bit smarter. Right at the end of an office visit, we started asking the parent who had come in that day which of them would be accompanying her the next time. A day or two before that next visit, that parent would be called and informed of the appointment. Even though it was a bit of a nuisance, our extra planning paid off. Despite the parent's communication problems, Francine remained on treatment schedule. Just when things started to become predictable, Francine's father got remarried. His new wife was a nurse and eager to play a major role in Francine's life. The new stepmother had very little, if any, knowledge about leukemia, but her nursing education made her think that she was an expert. Sometimes a little knowledge is truly a dangerous thing. The father's second marriage served only to worsen the already terrible communication between the parents. I ended up having to review information about Francine's condition and treatment at least twice in order to keep both parents well-informed. If Francine's mother was the parent who brought her to the office, then later that same day I would receive a call from her stepmother eager to know in detail what had transpired. Sometimes Francine's father would also call as he would not know that his new wife had already discussed the day's events with me. If her stepmother or father brought the child in for her visit, the situation was reversed. Usually the afternoon calls would include some snide remark about the other parent's lack of parenting skills.

Actually, I did not mind the extra discussions that much. At least they improved the communications. Within several months of starting treatment, Francine needed to be seen only once a month. I think that if her visits had been more frequent or complicated, I would have found the afternoon phone calls more of a problem. Almost one year after diagnosis and several months after Francine's father remarried, Francine's mother told me that her company was considering moving her to another state. She said she did not want to leave but wanted to be prepared in case she had to move. I contacted one of my colleagues near where she might be moving and arranged for him to assume Francine's care should that become necessary. Francine's mother asked me not to tell the child's father and stepmother about the possible transfer until the move became definite. At the time I thought it was nice of her to be concerned that her daughter's father and stepmother might be worried about a possible transfer which might not happen. As a result, I complied with her wishes. Once again I was naive. As it turned out, the transfer was definite. Francine's mother had not planned to tell her ex-husband and his new bride until after the move was completed. That way they could do nothing about it. Despite her attempts to keep the move quiet, the news managed to leak out. Francine's father called me about one month after I had learned of the transfer. He asked if I knew anything about the proposed move. I told him that I did not know for sure if the move was definite. I explained that I had made follow-up plans in the new city just in case.

His response was a plaintive, "But what about me? How will I ever get to see my children again?"

To be honest, my job description of physician does not include being a social worker or counselor, but I did feel very sorry for Francine's father. I imagined what it would be like not to be able to see my daughters because they now lived in another state. I could understand some of his anguish. Just because he and his former wife could not communicate did not mean that either of them was a bad or neglectful parent. Francine's mother was anxious to be free of the custody and visitation problems that divorce and living in the same city with her children's father and new wife had brought. She was sad about leaving me but felt that the change would be good for her and her son and daughter. Francine's father and stepmother were afraid that they were about to lose their involvement in the lives of the two children. The mother's job transfer was going to cause her and the children to move several states away. There was no way for them to stay as involved in the children's lives as they previously had been. They asked me to intervene. They wanted me to write a letter to the judge who had adjudicated the divorce saying that it would be dangerous for Francine to move to another state. The move would force the child to travel back and forth between the states several times each year so that both parents could retain their custodial rights. Francine's father and stepmother thought that they might be able to hold up the mother's transfer if I would tell the judge that such travel might aggravate the child's leukemia. Interestingly, Francine's mother was requesting that I use the exact same argument to keep the child from ever visiting her father again.

While there are definite things that are contraindicated for a child who is receiving therapy for leukemia, travel is not usually one of the dangers. I have had children mountain climb, ski, swim, run marathons and be involved in all sorts of activities while on chemotherapy. I made it clear to both sets of parents that I would not be used as a pawn in their game. I set up a meeting with both parents so that we could talk face to face about the problems that the mother's move was creating. I served as mediator and the two warring parents were able to reach a compromise of sorts. About two weeks later, Francine, her mother and her brother completed the move to another state and another treatment center. I continued to hear from Francine's mother on a regular basis. She would tell me what the new doctors were doing and she would then ask for my interpretation. It was uncanny. Usually the same day and just a few minutes after I heard from her mother, Francine's father or stepmother would also call. It was almost like nothing had changed at all.

A few weeks after leaving, Francine developed a serious infection. She required admission to a hospital for only the first time since the diagnosis of leukemia. This illness precipitated a crisis for her mother. She had established a strong sense of security with my management of her child, and she did not yet feel comfortable with the new doctors. During the first four or five days of Francine's ordeal, she would call daily or even twice a day. Finally, though, Francine began to improve and the calls came less frequently. The manner in which the new set of doctors had cared for Francine during the infection helped give her mother confidence in their skills. She began to call me less and less. A few months after leaving, Francine's mother remarried. Francine's father took an active interest in his stepdaughter's life, but I was not involved in any step- or biological-parent complications this time. For a few years I would see Francine every Christmas and sometimes during the summer, but she is now off chemotherapy and doing quite well. Her father and stepmother moved to another state almost five years ago and I have not heard from them since that time. Despite their divorce and obvious distaste for each other, both parents only wanted the best for Francine. Such is not always the case.

Vanessa's parents clearly thought of her cancer only as a means to satisfy their drug habits. Other parents habitually show up late or not at all for treatments or do not give medications necessary for the treatment of their child's cancer. Such cavalier behavior is always depressing and frustrating for the medical staff. It is impossible for those of us who take care of these children on a day-to-day basis to understand the motivation behind such parental neglect. Fortunately, the non-compliant parent is a relatively infrequent phenomenon. Most parents are actively involved in their child's care and will do anything to help him or her get well.

Divorce and remarriage create unusual situations for decision-making and support. Sometimes the parents are mature and communicate well for the sake of the sick child. Sometimes one parent does not stay involved in his or her child's life and does not know (or care) that his or her child has cancer. Sometimes both parents have remarried but retain joint custody and both think that each is the ultimate decision-maker. Under those circumstances, determining who is to make treatment decisions can be difficult.

Andy's family was the consummate example of the problems that such a situation can create. Andy was a pleasant 8-year old boy who had a malignant brain tumor removed from the back of his brain. Perhaps the family's difficulties stemmed from the fact that they had made extensive associations with the medical system earlier in Andy's life. Andy had been born prematurely and had gone through significant problems while still in the neonatal period. Following his birth at only 6½ months of gestation, he had needed to remain hospitalized for a prolonged period. After three months of innumerable tubes, IVs, tests and procedures, he had recovered and grown enough to finally go home. But he was not free of problems once he left the hospital. After his discharge, Andy had problems with poor weight gain and recurrent lung problems. These difficulties had necessitated frequent doctor visits. Andy had never gone more than two months without seeing a doctor or spending time in a hospital bed. It was ironic that when the brain tumor was diagnosed, Andy had been as well as he had ever been for more than a year. Because of the stress that had been brought on by his prematurity and the subsequent problems that he had endured, his parent's weak marriage had dissolved and both parents had subsequently remarried. The diagnosis of a malignant brain tumor forced Andy's parents to once again make significant medical decisions about their medically fragile child. Because of his parent's new marital status, the ease with which such medical decisions were made was significantly reduced. The two biological parents as well as the two stepparents felt that each had the duty and responsibility to make decisions how Andy would be treated. Andy's mother was the one who had official and legal custody, but she was uncomfortable making difficult decisions by herself. She welcomed the input of father, stepmother, stepfather, and all the other myriad family relatives who felt that they too should put their opinions into the mix. The neurosurgeon who removed the tumor had the easiest job. There was no doubt that the tumor had to be removed. This made it easy for the family to decide to proceed with surgery. Once the neurosurgeon had accomplished his task of removing the all of the tumor that he could see and Andy was beginning to recover from the surgery, he asked me to speak with Andy's family.

My goal was to educate the family about the type of cancer that had been found in Andy's brain and what treatments were available to try to keep it from growing back. Within a few minutes of meeting with the parents' family members, I realized that the two sets of parents actually had a different role for me in mind. They did not seem to want a physician who could help them with decision making. It appeared to me as if they were auditioning me for the role of pediatric oncologist. This made me very uncomfortable. I do not mind at all when a family seeks a second opinion. Frequently I find that a second opinion is a very wise and sensible thing to do. In fact, sometimes I am the one who suggests a second opinion so that I am sure that the care plan I have proposed is indeed the best for that particular child. However, I was very surprised and annoyed to find out that another pediatric oncologist had already seen Andy. The parents had already reviewed the diagnosis and treatment options extensively with this physician. I was quite unclear why I was being asked to see Andy. I found out about the second doctor by accident so that it was clear to me that the family had not wanted me to know about his involvement. What was the big secret? Who did they want to care for their boy?

The nature of that initial meeting enhanced the feeling that I was auditioning for this family. The first time I talked with the family, we met in a conference room about the size of an average school classroom.

Several chairs were arrayed in rough lines and scattered throughout the mid-sized room. There were no tables, lamps or bookcases to take up room or create a homier atmosphere. The chairs ranged from plush armchairs to simple stools. The various seats were filled with family members and curious onlookers whom I assumed were related to Andy or his family in some way. The four parents sat on comfortable chairs directly facing me. I sat center-stage in the middle of the room on a stool. The stool was made of wood and was the type that the class clown used to sit on when he was placed in the corner wearing a dunce cap when I was in grade school. Family members sat behind me and several others sat behind Andy's parents. Several more stood in the doorway in hopes of grabbing a few pearls of wisdom. The ages of the participants ranged from infants to grandparents. It was the largest audience I had ever had for a treatment-related discussion. At least sixty people crammed into the room. It was clear from the outset that father and stepfather disliked each other. It was also clear that they were best friends compared to the way that Andy's mother and stepmother felt about each other.

During the ensuing discussion, any statement made by one of the parents would be quickly and nastily dismissed by his or her unfriendly counterpart. This back and forth parrying and jousting quickly became tiresome. As thoroughly as I could, I discussed the possibilities and side effects of treatment. It was during this dialogue that I accidentally discovered that I was not the first to hold this sort of meeting with this family. Being asked to render a second opinion but not knowing that a first opinion had already been given did alter my view of the already bizarre situation. I tried not to let my annoyance show. I told Andy's parents that I favored using a newer technique for radiation therapy. I also suggested adding chemotherapy to the boy's therapy to try to give him a better chance for long-term survival. I made this suggestion because prior results using standard radiation therapy alone had resulted in dreadful outcomes with nearly all of the children with Andy's type of brain cancer dying within five years of diagnosis. I felt that those terrible results justified a much more aggressive approach. Whichever treatment was chosen, however, there were really no good second options should the first treatment failed.

The first pediatric oncologist who had seen the child had suggested that he be treated with the standard radiation therapy, since there was little evidence available to show that being more aggressive would actually improve the child's chances of being cured. I felt that either choice was truly appropriate based on the facts that were available to us. There are often reasons in medicine to choose different treatments for two patients with the same disease even though the two treatments may seem contradictory. One therapy might have more side effects but hold out the offer of a better chance of cure. The second option might be the more established treatment, but the outcomes with that therapy might be poor. Making such choices between treatments is always difficult. There are no clear answers or easy guidelines to follow. The family and the doctor must have an open, honest discussion of the facts, fears and realities. Time, patience and a caring attitude are necessary prerequisites on the part of the doctor. Review and re-review of the information are often necessary.

This decision, which may have life and death consequences for the child, is being made a very short time after the child has been diagnosed with a life-threatening cancer. The parents are still in shock and disbelief. Their ability to comprehend the nuances and subtleties of the various choices for treatment is often compromised. The decision as to which treatment will be used must be made and agreed to by both the parents and the doctor. The child, if he or she is old enough to comprehend the information and participate in the discussions, should also be asked for agreement to the decision.

Regardless of the decision made, it is important that the feeling be left that this important decision was made jointly by the doctor and the family so that no one shoulders the guilt alone should things go poorly. Guilt is a powerful emotion and rarely, if ever, deserved. I believe that whichever decision is made is the correct one as long as the people making the decision have carefully considered the facts and have made the choice out of their desire to do what is best for the child. In Andy's case, the bickering parents could not even agree which doctor to choose, let alone which treatment to select. It probably would have been better to have asked their divorce lawyers to mediate the decision. Somehow, those lawyers had gotten these bitter enemies to agree to terms of a divorce. At least, I think they had. I finally finished the marathon session and got up to leave. I was exhausted from the mental effort of trying to explain very delicate and sensitive issues in such potentially explosive surroundings. I asked one of the family members to contact me once they had reached a decision as to which doctor would be responsible for Andy's care. The next day I received the somewhat unenviable news that I had won the part. I guess I should have been honored, but I have never felt that caring for a child is a popularity contest. All I desired was that Andy should receive treatment from someone who wanted to provide the very best care for him. I knew the other doctor well and knew him to be fair, honest, caring and bright. I had no doubt that he would have done an excellent job for Andy. Instead, I had been voted "Dr. Congeniality" by a panel of judges. Selection of the doctor did not include a consensus agreement on the proposed treatment. For that, the family requested that all the doctors involved get together and make a decision. The family had concluded that they would abide by whatever decision was reached by the doctors. Since I had been selected as the physician of record, I had to contact the other pediatric oncologist so that together we could make a decision about which treatment to pursue.

Many children's cancer programs have established committees that review the cases of children who are newly diagnosed with some sort of cancer. These committees are composed of the doctors, nurses, radiation therapists, pathologists, nutritionists, physical and occupational therapists, surgeons, play therapists and other health professionals who will have a role in the care of the children. The available information about the child's cancer is discussed and a decision is reached as to which therapy would be best for that individual child. Sometimes the decisions are clear and easy to reach. Sometimes the choices are difficult and full of questions and unknowns. Andy's case fell mainly into the latter category.

After a lengthy and sometimes rancorous discussion between the nine physicians who were present, we decided that standard therapy would be used. I must admit that I was the major proponent of trying something new because of the poor results obtained with standard therapy, but I was overruled. Decisions rendered at a tumor board are not made based on any consideration other than what will be the best treatment for the child under consideration. All of the positives and negatives are evaluated and weighed. A tumor board offers the advantage of a thorough examination of the facts, a consensus opinion by the local experts and a diffusion of the feeling of guilt that making such difficult choices can bring. However, tumor boards like any committee, can be frustrating as they often lead pediatric oncologists to travel a route of compromise rather than risking the experimental or unknown path. Those who dare to take individual steps to try something new and untried are often the ones who innovate and improve on the current therapies. In taking chances, they take enormous personal responsibility and large professional risks.

I admire the innovators in medicine. They are the ones who have brought us so far in our fight against childhood cancer. I would love to report that Andy did better with the standard therapy than the children who had received it before him. However, nearly three years after the tumor was discovered and surgically removed, the cells reappeared. After an intense and prolonged struggle, Andy died from the cancer, almost exactly five years from the day he was diagnosed. My original impression of Andy's biological mother was that she had a weak personality and was easily manipulated. I was quite wrong. Once the original decision on how to treat Andy was made, she became the primary caregiver. She managed to keep the boy's father and stepmother almost completely away. Her passion for control became even greater after the tumor recurred. Because of her intense involvement and desire to keep Andy's father out of the loop, he did not get to see or help his son until just before his child's death.

Divorce and remarriage are just one of the ways that parental relationships may affect the care of a child with cancer. Sometimes the relationship between the parents can even color the way the child reacts to the treatments. I recall one child in particular for whom this was true. Chad was the oldest of three children. He was 16 years old when I first met him. He was one of the handsomest teenagers I have ever met. He was not, however, the least bit conceited about his handsome face or athletic build. He was very bright, modest, religious, warm and the boy most fathers would want their daughters to meet. He also was living under the cloud of having a slow-growing brain tumor in the center of his brain. The tumor had first been found when Chad was 9 years old. It was in a portion of the brain of major importance to mental functioning and so it had not been possible to remove it surgically. In order to control its growth, he had received radiation therapy and the tumor had stopped growing. The next six years had passed uneventfully. Chad was very popular at school and a role model for his younger brother and sister. At the age of 16, Chad was entering the prime of adolescence and showing promise for a successful and fulfilling life. Without warning, his plans and goals were shredded. Chad was in his high school English class presenting a report when he suddenly gasped, fell to the ground and began to thrash wildly about. His teacher stayed beside him while several classmates went to get help. None of them knew about his prior history. By the time EMS arrived, the epileptic seizure had stopped.

Chad was unconscious and unaware of his surroundings or what had happened. Still, his breathing was smooth and steady. He was rushed by ambulance to my hospital. The neurosurgeon who had originally made the diagnosis seven years earlier arranged for an emergency CT scan of the young man's brain. That study showed that the tumor was growing again. This was not all that unusual for the type of tumor that Chad had. These tumors often will lie quiescent following radiation therapy, but they are sometimes not completely subdued. Then, several years later and with little warning, they may begin to grow again. Regrowth can occur with amazing swiftness or it can occur subtly and slowly, but it is always unexpected. Regardless of how the tumor reappears, its re-emergence always signifies that the child's life will probably be cut short.

We all know that we cannot predict how long or how well we will live, but to be confronted with the capriciousness of life in such a way takes ones breath away. Chad's mother had invested her life and her love into her children, especially Chad. Chad was her special child. Perhaps that was because he was her first child and had taught her how wonderful being a mother was. Perhaps he had earned his place of honor in her heart because he was a unique child who was always obedient and sensitive to her needs and desires. She never could put into words what made him her favorite. He just was. Chad's father was proud of his son but not in the same way that his mother doted on him. He liked to go hunting with his son and enjoyed his companionship in a masculine way. Chad's father, however, was not a good communicator. He was definitely a sixties-type father in a nineties-type relationship. He felt that all it took to be a good father was to be a good breadwinner. To him, a father occasionally talked to his children about such subjects as sex, employment, hunting or fishing, but he needed to have little or no role in the actual rearing of the children. The women in his world were expected to be subservient to his needs. This is not to say that Chad's father was a caveman with no sensitivity to his wife or her needs. The two just happened to be on different wavelengths when it came to their marriage relationship. This would probably have been of little consequence if theirs had been the typical family from thirty years ago. Unfortunately, they needed to deal with a child with a recurrent brain tumor and to try to change a relationship that worked poorly most of the time but especially when times were tough. Chad had neither options for further surgery nor for radiation therapy. The tumor had recurred in the same place it had been before. Surgery was no more possible now than it had been when it had first appeared. He had already received radiation therapy and the surrounding normal brain would not tolerate more. Sometimes radiation therapy can be used a second time, but that was not the case for Chad.

Chad chose to fight his tumor recurrence with chemotherapy even though he was told that the chances of success were poor. Unlike many teenagers, Chad never asked why this had happened to him. Perhaps the seven years he had spent living with this tumor, silent but threatening, had allowed him to accept the unfairness of his situation. Losing his hair was somewhat difficult for him, since he had a model's hairstyle before the chemotherapy gave him a close shave. Still, he reacted mostly with humor rather than regret. He remained a popular figure in his school as well as in his small hometown. Everyone knew him and was rooting for him to do well. For a while, it appeared that the tumor was shrinking, but soon it started to grow again. Chad began to develop symptoms with the new growth that affected his ability to walk and talk. The tumor, however, never infected his spirit. He remained enthusiastic and continued to fight.

As it became more obvious that the tumor was winning the fight, we asked Chad what he would like to leave behind for his younger brother and sister. He really had no idea. We suggested that perhaps a videotape of his thoughts could be left to his siblings as a legacy. He quickly warmed to the idea. The next time he came to the office for a course of chemotherapy, a photographer was there to record his feelings and ideas. The videotaping was very moving and sad for those of us who were privileged to witness it being filmed. Chad looked directly into the camera and told his brother and sister that they must never give up no matter how difficult the tasks they faced. That message, delivered deep from the heart of a young man with every reason to give up, was passionate and inspirational. Few of us in and around his room that day remained dry-eyed.

Chad's mother could only react to Chad's illness with deep anger and sadness. At first, her anger extended to the doctor who had initially diagnosed her son's tumor. She felt that he had failed her and her son. In one way, he had. He had not allowed her son to outlive her. This was not his fault since the tumor had not been surgically removable either when it was first found nor when it recurred, but she had difficulty seeing this reality. Once she resolved her anger at the neurosurgeon, she directed her anger at her husband. Some of her anger was legitimate.

The entire burden of dealing with her son and his illness was left to her. She had to drive her child to every one of the treatments that progressively made him feel weaker and watch his suffering without having a shoulder to cry on at home. In many ways, Chad became her surrogate husband. He would talk to his mother about his feelings and then allow her to feel angry or sad or depressed without making her feel guilty for having those feelings. Chad also helped her cope with the behavior of his younger brother, Randy, who was 13 years old. This is an awkward and difficult age under the best of circumstances. Randy had already spent much of his short life trying to compete with his brother for his mother's attention. He had always felt that he was fighting a losing battle. He regarded Chad as some sort of perfect being and felt that he could never live up to his idealized image of his older brother. It was hard enough for Randy during the years that Chad was doing well. Chad would have been a tough act for any brother or sister to follow. The tumor, however, had served to further raise Chad's image. Chad had achieved a sort of martyr status. Randy felt that it was no longer even worth trying to compete since he would always come up short. In addition, Chad's treatments meant that the boy's mother had to pay even more attention to Chad. Acting out in school and insubordinate actions at home got him some attention from both of his parents, but not the positive approval he craved.

Randy's actions only worsened his situation. Some of his mother's anger began to be directed at him. Instead of the warm embraces he needed, he began to receive the brunt of her anger and bitterness. His father also reacted in a non-supportive manner. He had been feeling lonely and neglected because of his wife's increasingly tighter bond with her oldest child. Randy's actions only served to heighten his father's feelings of isolation and he projected these feelings onto the younger boy. Chad's sister was too young to be truly aware of all that was happening. She sensed the unhappiness that hung over the family like a miasma but did not know why. She was a quiet child and much younger than Chad so that Chad was more like a favorite uncle than a brother. His illness made little impact on her life other than to decrease the amount of attention she usually received from her parents. She had always been much more self-sufficient than her brothers had and so this loss of attention did not seem to be too significant to her. As Chad's condition deteriorated, so did the relationship between his mother and father. It reached the point where Chad's mother would not sleep in the same room with his father. He slept on the couch or at his office, which suited her just fine. Chad's mother turned to Marian for support as Chad's condition deteriorated. Marian served as the voice of reason at a time when the only thing that kept her going was emotion.

Finally, it became clear to even his mother that Chad was not going to get better. She decided that she wanted to care for him at home. Marian had established a close relationship with Chad and his mother and she stayed actively involved in his care. She often visited him at his home. Chad was delighted whenever she came. It was a sultry spring day when Marian made her first visit to the teenager's house. She was greeted effusively at the screened front door by his mother and directed into the house. The front door led into a nice-sized living room. A few days before Marian's visit, a hospital bed had been delivered to the house. Most of the furniture in the room had been pushed to the side so that there was room in the middle for a hospital bed. Since the young man could no longer provide for himself but was a fairly good-sized teenager, his mother needed the bed to help with his care. Chad's face lit up when he saw Marian walk into the room. He couldn't wait to show her his home. Almost as soon as she had greeted him hello, Chad pointed out the mounted head of a 12-point buck on the wall above the fireplace. With great pride, he told his visitor that he had been the one who had shot the whitetail. Marian did not understand that he was referring to the buck when he talked about the whitetail. Being a city slicker through and through, she thought that he was referring to a rabbit, since that was the only animal she knew which had a white tail. Chad roared with laughter when he finally caught on that she did not know that the buck was a whitetail deer. From then on, he never failed to mention her lack of country knowledge each time she visited.

Marian went to Chad's home three to four times each week. During his last week she was there every day. She was on her way to his home the day he died and arrived no more than 20 minutes after he drew his last breath. His mother was at his bedside holding his hand as Chad was released from his torment. The day he died was a beautiful early summer day. It was the kind of day on which Chad and his father used to go fishing and spend time together, but that was an earlier and more carefree time. Having Chad at home those last few weeks had allowed his mother to accept the reality of what was happening. When Marian came into the room on that day, she was silently crying, sitting at her dead son's bedside. After just a few moments, she noticed Marian's presence and stood up to hug her. The embrace was full of love and sadness and gratitude. Chad's father could do little. He clearly loved his son but did not know how to comfort his wife or his other children. He tried but had never learned how to express his feelings. When he did express his feelings, the feelings came out awkwardly. In reality, in that situation, it would not have mattered how eloquently he had expressed his grief. Chad's mother took out all of her anger at the senselessness of child's illness and death on him. She had shut him out of her grief weeks—and maybe even months—before her son had died. She had no intention of allowing him back into her life.

The boy's funeral was a special affair. The entire town turned out to honor the valiant teenager. Somehow during the funeral and the reception that followed, the family managed to project the image that they had been brought together by a common bond of grief. That image was clearly false. Chad's mother had shut his father out of her emotions and her heart. Her behavior was an attempt to move away from the horrible sadness and emptiness she felt. For a while she could not talk with her other children until Marian convinced her that they also were victims. They, too, had suffered from their brother's death. Now they had to endure not only their brother's death but also the loss of their mother's love and attention. Marian's words had an impact. Several months before Chad had died, it had been her desire to rent a motor home and drive through Colorado. Chad's illness had put that dream on hold. A few weeks after her son's funeral, she realized that she and the children needed to get away and she decided to take a trip to the mountains. While the aim of the trip was appropriate, the timing was not. The vacation proved to be too painful. Everything they did or saw reminded her of Chad. Then she would get angry with her other children because they were not Chad and Chad was never coming back. The only way she could move on was to discuss what had happened to Chad and to try to make some sense of it all. Somehow, with time and with Marian's supportive guidance, the relationship between the surviving children and their mother began to mend. Randy gave up his negative behavior and began to shine once his mother started to devote more attention to him. The youngest daughter, too, benefited by the change in her mother.

The relationship between Chad's mother and father, however, was shredded beyond repair. Years of non-communication and misunderstandings were wrapped up in anger over their child's untimely death. Within a few days of Chad's funeral, his father took his wounded feelings and sense of isolation into the arms of another woman. Even though she had rejected her husband earlier, this betrayal only further deepened his mother's feelings of anger and mistrust. She spent hours on the phone with Marian trying to decide what to do. She knew that she was desperately unhappy in her marriage, but Marian made her look at the practical consequences of divorce. Chad's mother had spent years as a housewife. She played the role of mother well but she had few marketable skills. Marian convinced her to take her time ending a long-standing marriage until she had a better alternative in its place. Chad's mother has slowly learned how to forgive and to make her life meaningful. While her children remain very important parts of her life, she realizes now that she must be a full person herself in order to provide the best for her children.

The lessons learned from a child's illness and death are often learned painfully, but can result in personal growth if one is willing to learn. Many people believe that the diagnosis of cancer in a child is a sure invitation to the end of a marriage. I have found that the diagnosis of cancer often makes a good marriage better. However, as it was for Chad's parents, having a child with cancer can often serve as the last straw to a marriage that is already weak.

As the years I have been in practice have passed, I have become more and more accustomed to seeing single mothers. Since most must work just to keep a roof over their heads and food on their tables, it is amazing to me that they can still find the time and the energy necessary to take care of their very ill children. Sometimes the divorced fathers have managed to have some ongoing involvement in their child's life. However, all sorts of interesting and difficult situations can result when the father decides to try to help out with the child's cancer care. Usually the father and mother have very poor communications even when it comes to the mundane issues that frequently arise in trying to raise a child in two separate households. Expecting the communications to improve when the two parents must deal with the complexities of cancer treatment is ludicrous.

The most common problems are missed appointments or medicines because one parent just happened not to tell the other when treatments were due. Other problems include housing and transportation difficulties as well as fighting between fathers and ex-mothers-in-law or mothers and the father's parents. Julie represents just some of the parental relationship problems that affect cancer care. Julie is now 13 years old. I became involved in her care just a little over one year ago.

Julie was living in a nearby town when she became tired and weak and began to bruise easily. She was seen by a local doctor who thought she might have leukemia. He called me and I agreed to meet the young lady at the hospital. I arrived at the hospital just a few minutes before the child was brought up to her hospital room from the admitting office. She was normally fair in coloring but her skin tone was so pale that she looked like she was made of alabaster. She was seated in a wheelchair that was being pushed by the admissions clerk. An elderly woman walked on one side of her. On the other side was another, younger woman who was very tall and who was crying and continually wiping a Kleenex over her running nose. Behind this group were a couple of men. Both were wearing baseball caps and t-shirts. Both looked bewildered and lost. Soon the girl was placed into her assigned room. I followed the entire entourage into the room to meet them and discuss the situation. When I asked who had been with her when she had been taken to the doctor, one of the men spoke up. He said that Julie had not been feeling well and so he took her to the doctor. A few more questions made it clear to me that this gentleman was not the child's father or her stepfather. It turned out the Julie's mother had been married three times. She was currently separated from husband number three and he was not present. Husband number two was Julie's father but he had very little to do with the child. Husband number one was the man who had spoken up. He had no blood relationship with Julie but he liked her a lot. She often would spend time with him especially when her mother had to work. It was fascinating to me that Julie was covered under his insurance.

Julie's mother could not stop crying. She was a hysterical sort of person and crying was her way of reacting to most situations. Her mother was the elderly woman I had seen when Julie was first admitted. Julie's grandmother was the main caregiver for the child when her mother or husband number one was not around. Julie's grandmother hated husband number one and he felt the same about her. Julie's grandmother wanted to know whether they could use the leukemia as a way to keep Julie from ever going back to husband number one's house, and whether there was someway we could ensure that husband number one would not drop the medical insurance he had on Julie. I do not enjoy dealing with such social questions.

I made it clear that all of the adults who were involved in Julie's life had to work together. Julie was my concern, not their petty differences. In spite of the potential problems raised by these very complicated relationships, they have managed to behave maturely around Julie. Her leukemia chemotherapy has remained on schedule. I think that this is largely because grandmother became the person responsible for making sure that Julie got all of her medicines. In fact, once Julie got better and left the hospital for treatment in the outpatient setting, I have seen her mother on only two occasions and have not seen husband number two or husband number one since. I have never met husband number three. I am glad though. I don't think I could keep all of the different relationships straight. Sometimes in a single parent home, the father (or mother) has left the scene completely and does not know or does not even care that his (or her) child has cancer. While such a situation is easier for me to deal with, I imagine that the involved parent must have great pain as a result. The situation is especially trying if the father or mother decide to re-enter the child's life—once diagnosed with cancer, after previously taking no part in the child's life.

One mother of a child who was newly diagnosed with cancer was so distraught that her ex-husband re-appeared (after essentially disappearing for several years) that she moved to another city. She gave me explicit instructions that I was not to tell the child's father where they had gone. Another time, a mother chose a false name for herself and her daughter so that her abusive ex-husband could not hunt them down. These types of situations are extremely difficult for the child, the parent who has accepted responsibility for the care of the child, the medical staff and me.

Divorce is never pleasant, especially when it involves children. It is even uglier when one or both of the parents decide to behave like little children themselves. Some single parents rely on other family members such as grandparents, aunts, uncles, older brothers and sisters, or even friends, to make it through the treatments. One mother had her next-door-neighbor bring her son in for his monthly treatments, since she worked and was afraid that she might lose her job if she took too much time off to bring her child to the doctor. Sometime on the day that her son was seen, she would call to find out how her son was doing and I would fill her in on the details. It was not a great situation, but it allowed her to keep her job and allowed me to continue to give her son good care. It must have worked because her child has been off ALL chemotherapy for almost three years.

Every now and then I meet a single mother (or father) of a child with cancer who is able to transcend the difficult situation through ingenuity and love for the child. Teresa was just such a mother. Teresa was a single mother who already had her hands full with two active teenagers. The older adolescent was a typical 15-year old girl who knew it all and knew that no one else did. She was positive that neither her mother nor her younger brother had any of the right answers. When Thomas, her younger brother, began to complain of dizziness and headaches, she was sure that he was just seeking attention. She only stopped teasing him when he became unable to walk. It became clear, even to her, that something was terribly wrong with her brother. Despite her outward appearance of non-caring, she truly loved him. She had a great deal of difficulty dealing with the reality that her brother had a malignant tumor growing in a small brain organ known as the *pineal gland*.

The presence of the pineal gland has been recognized since ancient times. The Greeks called the pineal the seat of the soul. Even today the function of this tiny gland is not clear. Some researchers believe that the gland may be important so that human beings can develop secondary sexual characteristics during puberty. Others feel that this tiny organ has some relationship to how we recognize light and darkness. Regardless of its function, the pineal gland can on rare occasions serve as the source of malignant brain tumors. The tumors that arise from this organ are often unusual. Why Thomas developed a malignant tumor in this mysterious brain organ is unknown.

After the tumor was identified and removed by the pediatric neurosurgeon, I was called to visit with Thomas and his mother. Thomas was 12 years old. He was scared—but also angry—that this tumor had happened to him. Despite being from a single parent family with no contact with his father for years, he was amazingly naive. Thomas's mother had been a single mother for four years. One day with no warning, Thomas's father had left for work and not returned. Even before he left, the times had not been pleasant. There were many evenings that Thomas and his sister had cried themselves to sleep because of their parent's violent fights. More than once the nights had been disturbed by visits from police called by neighbors to break up the warring adults.

Knowing that she would have to care for Thomas without the support of his father was not a source of discomfort for Thomas's mother. She was actually somewhat relieved that she no longer had to deal with the constant arguments and even physical abuse that had been a part of her life. She felt that dealing with her son's malignant tumor could not be any worse than what she had already faced and survived. Thomas's mother was a resourceful, bright, and hard-working woman who believed in self-reliance. She vowed to raise her children with love and good values, no matter how hard that might prove to be. She had a good job but decided that she could better herself by continuing her education. Her time spent studying served as a great role model for her children. They watched her working hard and tried to emulate her example. After graduating with a degree in business, Thomas's mother got an excellent raise in pay from the company where she had worked for eight years. When Thomas became ill, the pressure placed on her was immense. Her bosses relied on her and did not want her to take any time off. They told her that they were being supportive of her, but at the same time told her that her child's illness should not and could not interfere with her job performance. Still, right after her son was diagnosed and following his surgery, she took two weeks of earned vacation so she could sit at his bedside while he convalesced. Once he recovered from the surgery, the preteen was started on a combination of chemotherapy and radiation therapy.

The radiation therapy proved to be quite difficult for the young man. He received a treatment every day of the week, Monday through Friday. Saturdays and Sundays were rest days for the radiation therapy clinic and, subsequently, for Thomas as well. The harried mother would bring her child in for his appointment at the radiation therapy center at the latest possible moment. That allowed her to work most of the day. She would leave her office about one half-hour early, drive like a maniac across town to her apartment where Thomas was waiting. She would pick up her son and then race back to the other side of the town where the radiation therapy center was located. Her daily journey occurred just as rush hour traffic was almost at its peak so traffic was always hectic and congested. She would bravely and stoically battle the mass of cars each day so that they could arrive in time for Thomas to get his daily treatment. The treatments did not take long. Just a few minutes after arriving at the radiation center, she and Thomas would head out into the now crazy rush hour period to wage war once again with the tumultuous traffic. They would arrive home totally spent. The evenings were filled with getting dinner ready for her daughter and herself. Thomas usually did not feel well by the time they got home. Usually all his mother could get him to eat was a bowl of chicken broth. Once dinner was finished and the dishes cleaned and Thomas put to bed for the night, she would clean the house, do the laundry and pay the omnipresent bills before exhaustion finally overtook her. She would fall into a deep but often fitful sleep. Sometimes in the middle of the ride home or even later at night, Thomas would get sick to his stomach. After the first few experiences where she nearly joined her son in vomiting, his mother would travel the long journey to and from radiation therapy with a bowl and towel sitting on the floor of the car. Her experiences with Thomas made her a much more organized person. She learned how to be prepared for the most unexpected occurrences.

Thomas's sister did not cope as well as her mother with the marked change in the family's routines. The relationship between mother and daughter had not been good even before Thomas developed the symptoms that proved to be caused by the pineal gland tumor. Even though the mother had held her head high and kept the family together when her husband left, the teenage daughter had taken all of her anger over her father's abandonment out on her mother. Thomas's illness only gave her another reason to be angry. Tired from nursing her son and trying to deal with her job where she was given little slack despite her ill child, Thomas's mother had little energy left over for the almost daily fights and discussions with her teenage daughter. In order to make up for missing the last half hour of work each day, the harried woman would go in to work on Saturdays which gave her one less weekend day to recuperate for the busy week ahead. Her only pleasant times came on

Sunday afternoons, but only if Thomas felt well and if household chores were not too pressing. Even though the radiation therapy only lasted eight weeks, it seemed like an eternity to both Thomas and his mother. One Monday, while still getting radiation, Thomas, his mother, and his sister came into my office so he could have a blood count drawn and receive some chemotherapy. When Marian walked into the treatment room to draw the blood and to give Thomas his chemotherapy through his implanted central venous access device, his sister asked if she could watch. Thomas was afraid of the special needle used to access the implanted catheter. Whenever Marian came near him, he would flinch. His sister noticed his behavior and made a snide remark. Marian chose to ignore her until she was finished with the boy's treatment. When she had concluded, she turned to the young girl and asked her to join her in another office so that the two of them could talk. Marian has always had a way with teenagers. She knows how to reach out to them and find out their deepest concerns and fears. Thomas's sister was no different. The experienced nurse and the teenager had a long discussion in private.

Marian was able to get the young lady to see that her rude behavior was caused by her very real fear about her brother's well being. By the end of the session, she apologized to her brother for her lack of sensitivity. She even told her mother that she would try to be more helpful around the house. Marian suggested that the family would benefit from counseling so that they could continue to grow and realize how much they meant to each other. The whole family hugged Marian as they walked out of the office. Sometimes it takes a little active listening with a sympathetic ear to heal deep wounds.

Finally, radiation was completed. Thomas had lost nearly six pounds from his already too short and too thin body. Discussions began to center on how to improve his caloric intake. I was not surprised that Thomas had lost weight during radiation therapy. Radiation therapy takes a lot of energy out of a person and Thomas was no exception. Thomas had started out underweight so that the further weight loss was easily visible. The chemotherapy which would follow was expected to produce even further problems with the young man's already inadequate nutritional status. Thomas was only beginning to enter puberty. The weight loss further slowed his growth and development. He had little energy, was fairly irritable and depressed. Thomas tried to take special nutritional supplements but he hated the taste. After a few weeks of trying just about everything I could think of, I realized that Thomas needed more that what he could get in just by eating. I arranged for a special soft plastic tube to be placed through his nose, down his esophagus and into his stomach. Nutritional supplements could be given through the tube during the day and even at night without the boy tasting the materials. Within a week of starting (and despite his concerns about how he would look with a tube hanging out of his nose), Thomas began to regain some of the weight he had lost. The recovery was slow but steady. Soon he had lost his sunken cheeks and recessed eyes. His attitude improved dramatically as well. Watching Thomas made it very clear how much mood and good nutrition are interrelated.

Finishing the radiation therapy did not finish Thomas' treatments. With the completion of the eight weeks of daily radiation, Thomas now started courses of chemotherapy. The chemotherapy was given in six-week courses. On the first day of each six-week cycle, Thomas spent one entire day in the office with IV's full of chemotherapy medicines flowing through his veins. The chemotherapy made him sick to his stomach and caused him to lose his new found appetite. It would take him about one week to recover from that side effect. On the first day of the six-week period that the chemotherapy was due, Thomas' mother would take sick leave from her job and spend the day with him in the office. For the remainder of that week, he would be at home alone while his mother went to her job. She would call home every few hours to make sure that he was not having any problems. Her problems with her supervisors had not abated. They continued to warn the single mother that they would fire her if she missed any more work. The pressure on her to care for her child and yet maintain her source of income produced enormous stress.

The situation did not improve even after the wife of one of the supervisor's developed breast cancer. The supervisor could not understand why he needed to miss work since it was his wife who had the disease. Instead of making him more sympathetic, his experience actually made him more difficult. Fortunately, Thomas's sister did begin helping out a bit more as she recognized the terrible pressure being placed on her mother. The relationship between mother and daughter definitely improved, although it still remained bumpy at times. At least, they became more honest and open about their feelings and were more willing to share them.

Somehow, Thomas, his sister and his mother have made it through the treatments. Though initially feeling insecure and incapable of all that was asked of her, Thomas's mother has become a remarkably secure and self-assured woman. She can rightly be very proud of her accomplishments. She has raised two outstanding teenagers who have positive values and an optimistic view of life. They know that life can be very hard and can change at a moment's notice. They also know that hard work can often overcome many difficulties. Thomas is now in high school and his sister is in college. Their adventures in cancer were stressful but have made them both considerably stronger.

Although mothers are usually the main caregivers for their children, I have been impressed by the large number of fathers who take an active role in their child's illness. What has amazed me is that most of these fathers are very emotionally and passionately involved in their child's lives. I should not be so amazed since I am that sort of father. Still, the popular image of fathers is one of a stern, unapproachable, strong man who rarely, if ever, shows emotion. Many of the fathers with whom I have dealt are not like that. Many cry easily and do not consider a show of emotion unmanly. I have given and received many warm hugs from fathers over the years—hugs of grief, of joy, of fear and of fellowship—and I have never felt strange or out of place.

I learned a lot about fathers and their role in the care of their children early in my career from John. John and Kathy brought their son, Eric, to the hospital just after the local pediatrician diagnosed the little boy with ALL. In the space of two days, they went from being a very happy couple with a 5-year old boy and a second child on the way to a frightened pair of people in shock and totally unprepared for the diagnosis.

Eric did not cope well with his illness. He viewed the diagnostic tests and treatments as an assault. White coats and nursing uniforms became his enemies. He would scream long and loud whenever anyone in white entered his room. At first he was confined to his bed, but as his clinical status improved and he started to regain his mobility, his screaming would be accompanied by running away and hiding wherever he thought that he would not be found. Despite his efforts to become invisible, he was kept on therapy. After only one month of chemotherapy, he achieved remission.

Remission is an important step on the way to cure of leukemia and most solid tumors. Remission means that when doctors look at the person using standard techniques such as X-rays, blood tests, bone marrow examinations or spinal taps, no evidence of the malignancy can be found. Remission does not necessarily mean cure. Just because the tests do not show any evidence for malignancy does not mean that there are no cancer cells left behind. Techniques are not available to show every last cancer cell. It is felt that cure requires elimination of most, if not all, of the cancer cells. One cannot be cured of leukemia or cancer without first experiencing a remission, but being in remission is not a guarantee of a cure.

During the first few weeks of Eric's leukemia treatment, I got to know his mother quite well. Eric's father had to return to work shortly after bringing the sick child to the hospital. His mother was 5 months pregnant when her son became ill. The family only had one car and so the young mother had no ready means of transportation. In addition, both of the young parents had extended families who lived many states away and who could only visit during the first few days following the diagnosis. Eric remained in the hospital for two weeks after he was diagnosed with ALL before he recovered enough to return home. I should have suspected that a problem was brewing because once his father returned to work, he would call me every one to two days to ask how his son was progressing. He would preface his comments with the statement that he had no idea what was happening with his child. Each time he called, he seemed more anxious and angry, but I attributed that to his concern for his son. I did all that I could to reassure him that Eric was doing as well as could be expected. Eric completed the first month of chemotherapy without incident and easily achieved a remission. During the second month of treatment, Eric needed to receive two weeks of radiation to his head. The radiation was given to prevent the leukemia cells from finding a safe haven in Eric's spinal fluid where they could be protected from the chemotherapy. It had been known for a number of years before Eric was diagnosed that the spinal fluid represented a sanctuary for the leukemia cells. Late in the 1960's and early in the 1970's, it was discovered that it was extremely important to treat the spinal fluid as if it contained leukemia cells, even though none were seen on the diagnostic studies. Preventing the leukemia cells from recurring in the spinal fluid was a major breakthrough in the treatment of ALL. In those days, all children with ALL received radiation therapy to their heads as well as chemotherapy injected into their spinal fluids.

More recently, scientists have found that the radiation therapy can be safely eliminated from the treatment regimens of most children with ALL. The removal of radiation therapy to the head has been a good move since the radiation therapy was associated with learning difficulties, especially in very young children. It was also associated with an increased risk of brain tumors later after the leukemia was considered cured. Eric, however, was treated in the era when radiation therapy was still being given to every newly-diagnosed child.

Since Eric's family came from a far-off town, it was impractical for them to drive back and forth to receive radiation therapy each day. The Children's Hospital where I received my subspecialty training had a special unit where families could stay while their children were undergoing various treatments. The unit was designed as a place where families were taught how to care for children who had chronic medical problems so that the children could continue to do well once they were sent home. Each day I would come to visit Eric and his mother in their room on that special teaching unit. The instant I opened the door and Eric caught a glimpse of the white coat I had to wear as a fellow, he would scream in terror and run to the bathroom. During the first few days of his radiation treatment, he would lock the door and not come out until he was sure that I had left the room. As the days passed, he became less frightened by my visits. Towards the start of the second week of the radiation, he no longer would run into the bathroom. The screaming, however, continued. A few days before the radiation was completed, he was able to sit quietly next to his mother, though he would grab onto her dress hem like it was a security blanket. On the final day of that hospital stay, Eric actually talked with me and smiled at one of my silly jokes. It was nice that we had finally become friends.

About three months into therapy, Eric developed a fever. For most young children, a fever is a signal that their bodies are fighting off some sort of illness. Rarely is a fever dangerous. Children being treated for leukemia are different. The treatment of the leukemia weakens the child's ability to fight off serious infections. Sometimes a fever is the only sign that the child is very ill. When Eric's mother called to tell me that her son had a fairly high temperature and was lethargic, I told her to bring him immediately. His fever was indeed a harbinger of a serious infection and Eric had to be hospitalized. Eric's father dropped his mother and the sick boy off at the front door of the hospital. He could not stay. He had no more days off available to him and he would have lost his job had he stayed. The very pregnant mother held hands with her sick little boy as she waddled into the hospital lobby. A volunteer noticed them as soon as they entered and brought a wheelchair over. It took the volunteer a few minutes to realize that the chair was needed for the child. Soon the child and his mother were safely ensconced in a hospital room with IV fluids and antibiotics coursing into the child's veins. His mother sat in a comfortable chair at his side. She was clearly uncomfortable. No matter how much she fidgeted, she could not find a position that eased her discomfort.

Within a few hours of Eric's admission, his father began to call me. At first the father's voice was filled with anxiety and tension, but within a few days his tone became angry and hostile. Eric's father started to complain that his wife gave him no information about his son. He began to think that she was deliberately misleading him as to the severity of his son's condition since she seemed to have so little information. During this same time period, Eric's mother would pull me aside whenever I entered the child's room on rounds. She would express her anger and frustration at her husband for his lack of faith in her. She was bored, tired, anxious and frustrated. She wanted her child to get well and she wanted her pregnancy to be over. Adding to her resentment at her husband was her feeling of envy. Her husband was able to escape the constancy of the child's illness, but she was forced to confront it and deal with it each and every day. Eric's father expressed the exact opposite feelings. He was jealous that his wife could be at Eric's bedside and know everything that was happening to the child while he was forced to work at a boring, unfulfilling job that kept him away from the family he loved.

About two weeks before the new baby was due to be born and just before Eric had recovered enough to be able to go home, I arranged a conference for the parents so that I could communicate to them what I had observed. Both parents were confused, angry and anxious. Eric's father was furious that his wife could be with the child while he had to work. Eric's mother, on the other hand, was bored, tired and scared. She had to deal not only with Eric's illness, but also with feelings of malaise brought on by her advanced pregnancy. Neither was happy, and both were upset that what they felt was an ideal life was rapidly falling apart. I pointed out how they were directing the anger that they felt towards the leukemia at each other. Those feelings of anger were so intense that the couple was heading for divorce if they did not begin to pull together on the same team. I made it clear that they needed to use their energies to fight the leukemia rather than to fight each other.

Eric's mother, who had felt that her husband was lucky not to have to sit all alone in a dreary hospital room while trying to entertain a whiny, sick 5-year old hour after hour, was amazed to discover that her husband thought she was the lucky one. Her husband was equally surprised to discover that she thought that the fact that he could go off to work and escape the daily pressures brought on by Eric's illness was his good fortune. With the knowledge that they were both suffering and that they needed each other, they were able to work towards solutions and stop blaming each other for a situation which neither had caused. From these two parents I learned that illness in a child can lead to illness in a marriage. I was also able to see how deeply many fathers care for their children even when they cannot be directly at their sides.

When a child becomes seriously ill, different issues are raised than when a spouse gets sick. When either the husband or the wife develops a life-threatening illness, his or her mate can rally to provide the ailing one with support. However, when a child has a serious disease, both parents are in pain. At a time when both need each other's support, they are least able to give that comfort. Both parents may then feel neglected and turn their feelings of neglect into anger at the other partner. It is easy to understand how a marriage already under the strain of dealing with a sick child might shatter should those feelings of mistrust be allowed to fester. It does not happen often, but there are some families in which the father must take on the role of mother as well as father, breadwinner, and homemaker. Some of these fathers pay a high price for the "sin" of having a child with a malignant disease. Some have been demoted or lost their jobs. Others have lost relationships. The bottom line for these men remains that they do what they have to do in order to ensure that their children have their cancers treated. I admire them as well as the single mothers for their courage and determination. Some lesser people have left the child's care in the hands of relatives or even as wards of the state rather than face the difficulties produced by the disease and its treatment.

Rachel's father serves as a good example of one of these special fathers. Rachel was the first child I was called to see after I went into private practice. She was a 10-year old who had been diagnosed with a pineal gland brain tumor much like the one that occurred in Thomas. Rachel's parents had divorced many years earlier. Her father had remarried, but he and her stepmother had separated and were living apart just before Rachel turned ten. Rachel's father first noticed something was wrong with his child when he received a call from her schoolteacher. Rachel and always been a good student, but the teacher had noticed that the child was acting strangely in class. She was not finishing her work and she frequently complained of difficulty seeing the blackboard. When her father thought about it, he realized that he too had noticed changes at home. She was far more irritable. Her appetite was poor. She no longer wanted to go outside and play. He took her to a pediatrician who did a thorough examination. The pediatrician found signs of increased pressure on the young girl's brain. He quickly sent her for a CT scan.

A large tumor located in the center of her brain was easily visible on the X-rays. A local neurosurgeon had been reluctant to biopsy the mass. Rachel's father felt that a biopsy was necessary to know exactly what kind of tumor had been growing in his child's head. He drove 250 miles to the closest major city to seek out a neurosurgeon who would perform the biopsy. In less than one week after the discovery that the child had a brain tumor, the diagnosis of a malignant pineal gland tumor had been confirmed. The treatment selected was a very aggressive combination of chemotherapy and radiation therapy.

Within two weeks of diagnosis and surgery, the child had received her first course of intensive medications and had then been sent home to recover from the side effects. Rachel turned out to be very sensitive to the chemotherapy drugs. Her kidneys lost their normal function and became very leaky. Within days of returning from the distant city, the unfortunate girl became quite ill. Her father did not call the pediatrician who had obtained the CT scan since that doctor had not been told that the child had traveled to another city for a biopsy and treatment. Rachel's father was concerned that the pediatrician would be angry with him for not having his child treated locally. He did recognize that Rachel was becoming progressively weaker and so he brought her to the emergency room of a local hospital.

The emergency room doctor there was stunned by the condition of the child. He admitted her directly to the intensive care unit. Rachel was losing minerals and electrolytes vital to the function of her body at an alarmingly rapid rate. As fast as the IV's would replace the necessary materials, her kidneys would leak them out again. The emergency room doctor called in a kidney specialist to help with her care. The kidney specialist was uncomfortable dealing with the child since her kidney problems were due to treatment of a malignant brain tumor. He knew what to do about kidneys, but he did not know what to do with malignant brain tumors. That was how I got involved. Together we worked hard to correct the child's multiple problems. Slowly the treatments proved successful and she began to improve and regain her strength.

Rachel's father and stepmother had a rocky relationship almost from the day that they married. The girl's stepmother was a good woman who cared deeply about her stepdaughter. Despite the fact that she and Rachel's father were separated, she spent many hours at the child's bedside in the intensive care unit. Although she clearly cared for the child, she had two other children from an earlier marriage and so her focus could not totally be on Rachel. In addition, because of the circumstances of their separation, she was not completely comfortable around Rachel's father and he was almost always there. Thus it was left to Rachel's father to provide most of the girl's care.

Almost two weeks passed before Rachel had recovered enough to be ready to leave the hospital. On the day she was being discharged, I suggested to her father that she continue the chemotherapy with me. I was concerned about her receiving the treatment in one city and then getting severely ill in another. I did not consider this to be good care. She needed someone who was willing to take responsibility for her care following each course of chemotherapy. Rachel's father was at first reluctant to agree, but I promised him that I would follow the same treatment which had been prescribed in the other city. I am very glad that he agreed to allow me to continue his daughter's care. She did not have similar events like what happened with her first course of chemotherapy throughout the entire two years that the treatment lasted. Rachel and her father and I became very close over that time.

Chemotherapy medications are powerful drugs with potentially severe side effects. The margin of safety for these drugs is quite small and close observation is necessary. Even with very tight management, some children still develop problems. A certain number will require hospitalization for treatment of these problems and a smaller number will even die from them. Over the years during which I have been involved in the care of children with cancer, the intensity of the treatments has increased dramatically. More children have been placed at risk of side effects in an attempt to increase the overall cure rate.

The success story of childhood cancer and the increasing number of cured survivors have come with a definite price. The most common side effect produced by chemotherapy is a decrease in the white blood cell count. The white blood cells are very important in fighting infections. A decrease in the number of white cells that are available can produce an increased risk that the child will develop a serious infection. About half the time that the white count becomes very low, the child will develop a fever. Most often they will then need to be admitted to a hospital and given intravenous antibiotics. Once the blood count improves, the fevers usually disappear. Once in a while, severe or even life-threatening infections may occur. Rarely, those infections prove fatal. Rachel's father was very grateful that the doctors in the other city had diagnosed the tumor. He had great faith in those doctors despite Rachel's initial nearly fatal reaction to the chemotherapy.

Once a week even after I took over the actual care of the child, he would drive the 250 miles to the city where treatment had been started. The drive was long and tiring. Rachel was angry when they left and sick when they returned. Rachel's father had no choice but to take large chunks of time off from his work in order to take his child to her therapy. The patience of his bosses, which had not been great even before Rachel first became ill, wore progressively thinner until he was finally laid off from his job. The loss of his job was even more devastating since he also lost the health insurance that had covered his daughter. Because she had a brain tumor, she had essentially become uninsurable.

Recently passed legislation, such as the Kassabaum-Kennedy bill, hopefully will decrease or even prevent such problems from occurring, but such measures were not available for Rachel and her father. Fortunately, although Rachel might no longer have been covered by insurance, but she did not lose any of her access to the care that she needed.

Rachel and I developed a close relationship in those early days. No matter how sick she was, I was always able to make her laugh. When I first met her, her arms could not easily move since she had intravenous lines in both of them. She would tell me that was all right by giving me the 'great-toe up' sign. When I saw her raise her foot and extend the great toe, I knew all was well. After a few days of watching her signal her status to me, I began taking off my shoe and giving her a great-toe up sign in return. That response has remained our own personal signal that all is right with the world. Just recently, nine years after her diagnosis, Rachel came to visit me to get some information she needed for a college class. In the middle of the hallway of the medical office building, we both took off our shoes, gave each other the great-toe up sign and then giggled. Only someone who has gone through the experiences that Rachel and I shared could understand the deep meaning behind our signal.

The support and love that Rachel's father gave to her was unconditional and gentle. The generalization that men are non-supportive, non-communicative and unable to give of themselves does not apply to most of the fathers whom I have been privileged to know.

The Medical Road I Travel

The road that I have traveled the past 20 years has been full of magnificent landscapes and wonderful events, but also has been pitted by potholes, assorted detours, unexpected turns and twists. I am happy I have gone on this journey in spite of the many times I have had a great desire to turn around or to take what appeared to be an easier byway.

Through the years, the technology with which I have traveled has improved and changed. Much of the improvements have occurred because of the work of some amazing and dedicated physicians and nurses. Just 50 years ago, a diagnosis of cancer in a child was nearly always a death sentence. If the cancer could not be removed with surgery or treated with the limited forms of radiation therapy then available, there were virtually no survivors.

A major advance occurred in 1955 with the establishment of the Children's Cancer Group. This organization was started by eight forward-thinking pioneers in the field of childhood cancer. These physicians realized that there were not enough cases of childhood cancer at any one center to do the studies necessary to improve the lot of a child with cancer. They decided that there must be cooperation between institutions for the betterment of all the children. The unique structure they established has grown into the world's largest network of doctors, nurses, and other health care professionals dealing with the problem of childhood malignancies. The success of the Children's Cancer Group and of a second group established several years later, the Pediatric Oncology Group, is nothing short of miraculous. Nearly 3 out of every 4 children diagnosed with cancer today are expected to be cured of their disease. For some kinds of cancer, the results are even better. For some, such as brain stem gliomas and neuroblastoma, much more work remains to be done.

The treatment of childhood cancer has proven to be much more than dealing with the cancer itself. A child with cancer is part of a family greatly affected by the disease. In turn, the family affects the outcome of the child by its attitude and involvement. The child has to grow and develop and at the same time fight a particularly difficult foe. This makes the child much different from the adult who develops cancer. Sometimes the social, psychological and emotional burdens placed on the family and the child by the cancer are worse than the cancer itself.

In this book, I have tried to use examples of patients I have worked with through the years to demonstrate and describe some of the emotional, physical, spiritual and psychological events that affect a child's cancer experience. I want to describe two children whom I think provide a final insight into the dilemmas and difficulties that a children's cancer doctor faces when dealing with these children.

Andrea had turned 6 years old just two days before she was diagnosed with ALL. The findings of her blood count and her age suggested that she had a very good chance of being cured. She was started on chemotherapy within a day of presenting to the hospital and her initial response was quite gratifying. The leukemia cells seemed to melt away before our eyes. In less than one week, she was ready to go home.

Being ready to go home did not mean that she was entirely safe. The bone marrow quickly emptied out many of the leukemia cells, but there were no normal cells to take their place. That would take a few more weeks. Still, it was safer to have her away from the hospital with all of its potential germs. Andrea was sent home with several medicines and her parents were warned to call for any problems, especially fevers.

About half of the children who go home shortly after beginning therapy for ALL have to come back to the hospital because they develop some sort of problem, most often fever with no obvious site of infection. Andrea was in that half of patients. One morning three days after she arrived home from the hospital, I received a call from her mother. Andrea had spiked a temperature to 102° F. She otherwise had no other signs of infection.

Andrea and her mother arrived at the hospital within an hour of that phone call. An IV was started quickly and blood cultures were drawn to see if we could identify a bacteria or fungus that might have been responsible for the fever. As we expected, her blood count showed her to have very few of the white cells necessary for effective response to infections. Within 2 hours of the original call, labs had been obtained and fluids and antibiotics were flowing into the veins of the little brown-haired girl.

I met the child and her mother when they arrived at the hospital. The child was in good spirits in spite of her fever. Her only complaint was that she felt a bit tired. My examination did not reveal any source for the fever, but that was not unusual under the circumstances. Most of the time, no source is ever found for the fevers that occur when the white blood cell count is low. The antibiotics that are selected are designed to cover a wide variety of possible infections since many germs which are normally not dangerous can cause serious problems when there are not enough white cells.

About two hours after I examined Andrea and explained the situation to her mother, I received a call from her nurse. He was concerned because the child's blood pressure was several points lower than it had been when she had arrived at the hospital. I ordered the nurse to increase the fluids that Andrea was receiving in her IV and I headed back to the hospital.

It took me only about 30 minutes to get to her bedside but by the time I arrived, Andrea was in full-blown shock. Her blood pressure was quite low and her heart was racing. She was quite pale and her fingernails were bluish in color. An oxygen mask had been placed over her face, but she was gasping for each breath. Her eyes were filled with panic. Her mother gripped her hand and tears rolled down her cheeks.

Knowing I could not arrive there right away, the nurse had called the *intensivist* as soon as he had hung up the phone with me. An intensivist is a specialist in the care of children in the Intensive Care Unit. The intensivist had already ordered medicines to support the child's falling blood pressure. Once she was stable enough, she was rapidly moved to the PICU. Monitors were strapped into place to measure her heart activity and her oxygen level. Within moments of arriving, a tube was placed through her mouth into her airway so a machine could do the work of breathing that had become so difficult for her. Soon there were tubes and catheters running from several sites. It has always amazed me how quickly a child can go from looking normal but not feeling well to a heavily sedated being on a mechanical respirator with tubes seemingly coming out of every orifice. If I am amazed by that, I am sure the families are dumbfounded.

I left the PICU once I had confirmed that the situation was as stable as possible and that Andrea's mother had been told what had happened. It appeared that Andrea's fever did have a source. The rapid downhill course suggested that Andrea had a bacteria in her blood. When the bacteria had suddenly been exposed to the antibiotics, toxins were released by the dead bug. The toxins had caused her blood pressure to plummet. Despite our attempts, no bacteria were ever grown from Andrea's blood.

I returned to the PICU that evening to check on the child. Her blood pressure had not varied a lot once it had been stabilized with the medications given to her by the intensivist. Her pulmonary status was good on the respirator. She did not look better but at least her condition had not worsened.

I arrived in the PICU the next day with a great deal of anxiety. I had received no calls during the night, which was good news. Still, I knew that the intensivist was doing most of the work and would have received most of the calls from the nurses. The intensivist who had been there all night was ready to leave, but he expressed some optimism about the child's situation before he left for the day. That was encouraging. Usually shock due to a bacterial infection occurs quickly and the clinical course often goes rapidly downhill. The fact that Andrea had survived the night and seemed to be a bit better as dawn approached was reason for encouragement.

The path of improvement seemed to be as swift as the path downward had been. Within another day the respirator was withdrawn since she was breathing easily on her own again. Soon all of the tubes and gadgets that had been so necessary just a few days earlier were also taken away. Andrea had returned.

Andrea completed chemotherapy for ALL a little over two years later. Her course was benign from the moment she left the PICU. It has now been seven years since that horrible episode and Audrey remains an honor student with a caring and warm personality. She does not remember at all what happened, but her parents and I still recall it vividly. Andrea clearly represents one of the great triumphs of a children's cancer doctor.

Ricky, however, points out the other side of this field that makes it so difficult for many people to appreciate how far we have come in the past 40 to 50 years. Ricky was a vivacious, towheaded 16 month old. His parents had struggled with infertility problems for years before he was born. He was the first grandchild on either side of the family and he brought the loving family even closer together.

The small family had established a tradition of visiting the father's parents in Indiana every summer. On the plane ride there just a few weeks before I met him, he had not wanted to eat and had been irritable. His parents thought his behavior was due to a reaction to flying, but the toddler continued to be irritable even after a few days at his grandparent's house. When they noticed that Ricky's belly was getting bigger and there was something firm on the left side, the family visited a local doctor. The doctor reassured them that it was just the strange environment that was causing Ricky to be out of sorts. In addition, he thought the firmness in the abdomen was due to constipation.

When the family returned home several days later, Ricky continued to be irritable. His parents brought him to his regular pediatrician who felt the abdomen and noted a large mass. The mass was not due to constipation. The pediatrician ordered a CT scan. By the next day, she knew that the mass was very large, filling up most of the left side of the abdomen. It appeared that the tumor mass arose from the adrenal gland sitting just above the kidney. It stretched up to the diaphragm and pushed the stomach and intestines toward the right side. It not only had grown upwards in the abdomen but also downwards as well. It had surrounded the left kidney and was blocking the drainage of urine from that kidney into the bladder.

The size of the tumor was astonishing since Ricky had been eating normally and having few complaints until a few days earlier. I received a call from his pediatrician within moments after she found out the CT scan results. Within two hours, Ricky was in a hospital bed and the evaluation was proceeding. The studies showed that the tumor had spread into some lymph nodes in the boy's neck, but they showed no evidence of tumor elsewhere. The tumor in the abdomen could not be removed since it was invading around the all of the major blood vessels and organs. It was decided that the best way to get tumor for biopsy was with a needle placed into an involved lymph node in the neck. It took only two days for us to find out that the tumor was a neuroblastoma.

A neuroblastoma is a tumor that arises from the sympathetic nervous system. The sympathetic nervous system is sometimes called the involuntary nervous system. The source of Ricky's tumor was the adrenal gland, an important gland that sits on top of the kidney. This tumor is one of the most common solid tumors seen in childhood. It occurs most often in very young children. In those over a year of age at diagnosis, the prognosis tends to be poor if the tumor has already spread when it is found. Since the tumor tends to spread very early, 70 to 80% of the tumors have already spread to other tissues by the time they are diagnosed. Even with the most aggressive therapies, only 35% of the children with the most advanced form of the disease survive without any evidence 3 years following diagnosis.

That was what Ricky faced. It was essential that chemotherapy be given to try to shrink—and hopefully eliminate—the obvious signs of the tumor. Even if the tumor could be completely eliminated, he would still have to undergo a bone marrow rescue procedure using his own bone marrow cells. All of this information was laid out for the little boy's parents. They sat in stunned silence and wondered how this disaster had ever happened. There were no good answers since the cause of the tumor remains unknown. The parents felt they had little choice. If they did not proceed with treatment, the tumor would continue to grow and he would die of the tumor. If they did go ahead, he might respond and might have a chance at survival, but the treatments had their own potential toxicities and side effects which made the prospect of therapy less than appealing.

The next day Ricky started chemotherapy. For the first four days, he did fairly well. His abdomen remained distended and hard. Then a big change occurred. Ricky's abdomen became even more distended and firm. It stuck out so much that the surface was shiny and tense. Ricky's blood count showed a significant decrease in his red blood cells. The results suggested that the tumor had ruptured open and was bleeding into the abdomen. Ricky began having trouble breathing because the very firm abdomen was pushing his diaphragms up and compressing his lungs. There was little room left for the lungs to expand and fill with air. As with Andrea, Ricky was soon in a room in the PICU with a tube in his throat attached to a respirator and tubes and lines running from many different sites to various monitors and pumps.

Within a few hours, it became clear that we had a serious dilemma. In order to stabilize the child's blood pressure and improve his condition, emergency surgery was necessary. However, entering the abdomen under such precarious conditions would cause release of quite a bit of blood which was undoubtedly under some pressure. When the blood was released, it was highly likely that the tumor would start to bleed again. There was a great concern that it might not be possible to stop the bleeding. The surgeon and I spoke with the anguished family at length. Together we chose to take the child to surgery. Within an hour the child was being wheeled down to the operating room. I had no role to play in the surgery, but I wanted to be there anyway. I put on surgical scrubs and proceeded to the operating room.

With great care but with appropriate speed, the surgeon proceeded to open the abdomen. As soon as the scalpel passed through the final layer of the abdominal wall, blood came spurting out. Soon enough blood had been drained from the wound to replace the child's blood volume two times over.

The surgeon continued to look into the open abdomen. Tumor was everywhere on the left side. All he could do was take a surgical spoon and scoop out some of the excess. He then began to pack the area where the tumor had been bleeding with materials to help the area clot. Finally it seemed the bleeding was under control and the abdomen was again closed up. Ricky was moved to the PICU to recover. That night was very difficult for the family and for me. Would he continue to bleed out from the tumor or had the surgery controlled the hemorrhaging? By morning it appeared that the bleeding had stopped.

Ricky's problems were far from over. The bleeding the day before had caused his blood pressure to drop a bit from the high values he had exhibited when he had entered the hospital. During the night following the surgery, the blood flow to the lower half of his body had decreased.

The intensivist had used many different medicines to try to get the blood pressure to increase and to improved the blood flow. His efforts had been somewhat successful, but by the next morning the infant still had cold legs and evidence of decreased blood flow.

Despite the surgery and Ricky's critical condition, the chemotherapy continued. A few days after the emergency surgery, it became obvious that the tumor bleeding had stopped. It also became obvious that Ricky's kidneys had been damaged by the period of decreased blood flow that had preceded and followed the surgery. They were putting out very little urine. The waste products normally removed by the kidney were being retained. Kidney dialysis was started to try to clear the blood of excess fluids and waste products.

The abdomen remained distended, which prevented Ricky's lungs from expanding fully and he required the respirator in order to breath and maintain his oxygen level. The chemotherapy drugs began to cause a decrease in the production of bone marrow cells. Ricky's blood cell counts started to decrease significantly. After a few days, he developed a fever and was started on antibiotics to fight any potential infection. His kidney's continued to worsen until he finally stopped making urine altogether.

After two weeks in this condition his parents finally asked a very important question: what was the chance that he would improve enough to get another course of chemotherapy? A repeat CT scan did not show any change in the size of the tumor. It would be extremely difficult to give chemotherapy while he remained on dialysis and his condition was such that most people would not even consider a bone marrow rescue (which was clearly necessary in order for him to be cured of the original tumor). His parents did not want him to suffer, but they also did not want him to be kept alive by machines if there was no chance he would improve.

The parents and I decided together to try to verify whether Ricky's kidneys would ever recover. I felt that he had to have working kidneys in order to get better from all of the problems afflicting him. We chose a study that would not cause a great deal of pain or distress to the child. It showed that there was some blood flowing to the kidneys, but there was no evidence that his kidneys had any function nor that they would they ever function again.

There was little cause to continue with support. All we were doing was prolonging the child's death. We were not doing anything to improve his chances of living. A conference was held with the parents, the grandparents, the family pastor, the intensivist, the nurse who was currently on duty and myself. In a very open and honest way, we discussed the situation and the various options. The conversation was painful and difficult. A great many thoughts and ideas were reviewed, but finally it was decided to withdraw much of the supportive medicines and machines that were keeping Ricky alive.

There was a great deal of concern that if the respirator was withdrawn, the child would gasp and struggle for air. This would be very distressing to his parents and to the medical staff. As a result, the respirator was not withdrawn immediately. With his kidneys no longer treated with dialysis, Ricky's condition remained fairly stable. He became somewhat puffy because the dialysis was no longer removing excess fluid. Ricky's parents, grandparents and the family pastor said a prayer at the child's bedside and gave him a final good-bye kiss. The scene was emotionally draining and terribly poignant. Every one of the medical staff personalized the situation. How would they have felt if Ricky were their child? Would they have been able to agree to stop the therapies? Would they be angry, feel cheated, sad, overwhelmed with grief? Finally, the family was ready and the respirator was disconnected. Within a few moments, it became clear that Ricky was unable to breath on his own without the ventilator support. He quickly turned blue and his heart rate and blood pressure rapidly dropped. Despite the changes, he did not gasp or appear in any pain or distress. His mother held him in her arms as he took his last breaths. She caressed his head and his father kissed him as he gave up his fight for life.

Ricky's case was agony for his parents, his grandparents, the intensivist, the nurses and for me. Did we go too far to try to save him? Did we do too much? Did we do enough? There are those who would criticize the choice made by the medical staff and the parents. Sometimes advances in medical technology can sustain the appearance of life but not life itself.

It is my fervent hope that advances that will continue to be made will allow children's cancer doctors like myself to deal only with the triumphs and never with the tragedies. Until then, we must continue to face these very difficult situations and complicated questions with knowledge, sensitivity and a deep sense of caring. Together, we will be successful at conquering kid's cancer.

What Parents Can Do

Parents can enhance their child's care in many ways. Here are just a few of them, gathered from years of observation and participation:

Stay involved. If you are the primary parent, go to the doctor's office as often as possible. If unable to be with your child, call the doctor or nurse for an update.

Become knowledgeable. Few people know much about children's cancer when their children are diagnosed. Usually very little information is retained from that time. Once the shock of the diagnosis has lessened and treatments have become routine, begin reading and learning more about your child's disease. There are many resources available including your doctor or nurse, the Leukemia Society, The Brain Tumor Society, the American Cancer Society, the library, the Internet. In addition there are several support groups including the Candlelighters and specific disease oriented support groups that can serve as excellent sources of information.

Become aware of your child's treatment protocol. Most children are treated according to a protocol developed by one of the major children's cancer treatment groups. These protocols have specific phases and guidelines. Most programs will be able to provide you with a daily calendar of what medicines your child should be receiving. You should also have a list of possible side effects to expect from each medicine. Learn what medicines your child should be receiving and what they look like. Keep the doses written down. Your doctor and nurse are responsible for many children and can make mistakes. You are responsible only for your child. If you know the medicine and the dose your child is to receive, you can verify that what your child is receiving is correct.

Keep your child's teachers and counselors aware of your child's condition. Many programs will have school reentry programs which are designed to make your child's return to the school environment much easier. Discuss your child's condition with the teacher often. Watch out for problems and head them off before they occur. Some teachers think that children with cancer are always sick and cannot learn and so the children end up receiving an inadequate education. Some teachers are not very compassionate and do not make allowances for the child's disease. The child may then end up suffering as a result.

Write down prescription information so that medicines can be given correctly. There is a very narrow margin of safety for most of the chemotherapy agents. Giving too much at one time can result in undesirable or even dangerous side effects. Giving too little can allow the cancer to grow back. It is difficult to remember verbal instructions, even when they are repeated several times. Write down the instructions in a journal. Use a daily pillbox and place the necessary pills in the appropriate box for an entire week or even an entire month. It is best if at least two people in the family are aware of the treatment plans and the dosages so that the correct medication amounts and types can be confirmed. If in doubt, call the doctor or nurse.

Do not be afraid to contact the doctor or nurse. There are many questions which arise regarding day to day activities. No matter how thoroughly you have reviewed all the possible events with your doctor or nurse, things will happen that will not be anticipated and that may affect your child's care. Pick up the phone and call. It is highly likely that the medical team has dealt with your child's problem before and knows what to do. Sometimes the question will lead to a change in plans that will greatly impact your child's care. Do not wait for a few days to find out what will happen. Call when the problem arises. Nothing is more frustrating to a doctor or nurse than to find out that there is a problem that could have been dealt with but the time to correct the problem has passed because the parents did not call.

Be assertive but not aggressive. Anger, frustration and fear are common emotions for parents whose children have been diagnosed with cancer. Some parents react to such emotions by becoming demanding, bossy or interfering. Such reactions can strain the relationship between the medical staff and the family. Try to remember that the medical staff is on the same team and is working for the same goal. If you do need to express anger or disappointment, do so in private. People can change their behavior when it is pointed out to them, but they will not if they are placed in a defensive position. **Let extended family members help.** Grandparents, uncles and aunts, cousins and others can be of great help. They can give breaks to weary parents, give moral support, or even take the children to medical appointments (or spend the night with the children in the hospital). Do not be a martyr. Caring for a child with cancer is a major undertaking and support is always welcome. Be careful, though, of unwanted medical advice. Often, family members will make medical suggestions based on very little information. While they are well-meaning, this medical advice is often erroneous or misleading. It is also being given at a time when the parents are most vulnerable to any suggestions. Recognize that the person who is offering the advice is only trying to help. Let them know you appreciate their thoughtfulness but also let them know that you already have knowledgeable doctors caring for your child. Those who specialize in this field have access to information from all around the world. They choose a treatment for a child because it truly is the best treatment for that child.

Continue to provide discipline and guidance for your child. There are few things worse than a child who uses the cancer and its treatment to get away with inappropriate and bratty behavior. At our office, we have placed children in time-outs and had firm discussions with the parents in order to correct behavior that not only alienates the medical staff but may endanger the child. We do not allow kicking, screaming, biting or other destructive behaviors. Children need to have boundaries on their behavior and discipline so that once the cancer is cured, they can grow up to be responsible and mature adults.

What Medical Personnel Can Do

Doctors and nurses may do many things to enhance the care of the children. Here are the most important and obvious ones:

Listen to the parents and the children. The parents know their child better than you ever will. They can often recognize subtle changes in behavior and demeanor that have important implications.

Address the parent's concerns. Do not dismiss a parent's concerns about their child as foolish or uncalled for. Parents come from a variety of different medical and social backgrounds that affect how they view their children and their illness. Just because their views and concerns do not match yours does not mean that those concerns are not valid. Try to address not only those concerns which are overtly expressed but also those which are implied by the parent's body language or tone.

Never yell at or criticize a parent for being concerned. Regardless of the nature of the call or question, always make the parent feel that their concern is appropriate and timely. Once the parent's specific concerns are addressed, it is appropriate to educate them as to what your concerns are and why.

Be sincere. If there is bad news, take the family to a quiet, private area and make sure that you are not disturbed. Sit down with the family and don't be afraid to let them know that you are upset or affected by the bad news. Parents accept news much better when they know that the medical personnel have a personal interest in what happens to their child.

Be honest. If a mistake has happened, let the parents know. Do not cast blame onto others or try to escape responsibility for what has happened. Parents usually appreciate knowing that doctors are human beings.

Be knowledgeable. It is not possible for anyone to know everything. In difficult situations, be willing to let parents know that you have contacted outside resources for additional information. Do not be afraid to offer to send the child for a second opinion if you feel that the parents or child will benefit from another doctor's experience or knowledge. Your ego will not cure the child.

Do not become enamored by your title. Your license gives you the right to practice medicine but medical knowledge is not divinely imparted. It is very difficult to work with a doctor who is arrogant and full of him or herself. Remember that the care of children with cancer is very much a team effort and requires the input of nurses, social workers, dieticians, other doctors, physical and occupational therapists, play therapists, clergy and others.

Give a single, clear message. During the initial diagnosis and throughout their treatment, the families will come into contact with a large number of medical professionals. Each will give the family some knowledge about the child's disease. Since each professional has different experiences, the message given to the family may be different and confusing. It is important that the parents easily recognize and identify the doctor who oversees care. That doctor needs to do all he or she can to dispel confusion.

Be available. Do not hide behind a phone system or in your office. Make yourself available in person and on the phone. One of the greatest frustrations for a parent is to not be able to reach the doctor or have the doctor return the call. This is particularly true when the parent is waiting for the results of lab work or of X-rays. In most cases, results from tests come back very soon after the test is completed. There should be no reason to make parents wait several days or even weeks to have the results made available. You would not want that done if it was your child. Why do it to someone else?

Be pleasant. There is nothing to be gained from rudeness or being abrupt either to parents, children or to fellow medical personnel. Even when frustrated, a positive attitude tends to get things done quicker and more efficiently.

Don't be afraid to give of yourself. Somewhere medical schools have been taught the message that it is dangerous to feel compassion about your patients. It is important to maintain objectivity, but it is okay to allow your feelings to be expressed. Parents really appreciate knowing that their child's doctor has feelings and cares. It gives a sense of security.

Ask others for help and advice. No one can succeed alone and many others genuinely want to help. Let them help when appropriate and possible.

Keep yourself heathy and happy. A good example is undeniably good for others to see and emulate. Your judgment will be better and so will your attitude, your demeanor and your strength for those short of hope.

Organizations

American Cancer Society

1599 Clifton Road NE
Atlanta, Georgia 30329
(800) 227-2345

American Brain Tumor Association

2720 River Road, Suite 146
Des Plaines, Illinois 60018

**Candlelighters Childhood Cancer Family Alliance
(Candlelighters Childhood Cancer Foundation)**

7910 Woodmont Avenue, Suite 460
Bethesda, Maryland 20814-3015
(800) 366-2223
info@candlelighters.org

Leukemia Society of America

600 Third Avenue
New York, NY 10016

National Childhood Cancer Foundation

P O Box 60012
Arcadia, CA 91066-6012

See the website and many varied links

http://www.emeraldink.com/children.htm

E-mail the author

kidscure@flash.net

GLOSSARY

Absolute Granulocyte Count (also called ANC)

Multiplying the total number of white blood cells times the number of granulocytes (segs + bands). For example, if the overall white blood cell count is 5,000 and there are 50% granulocytes, the absolute granulocyte count is 2,500 (5,000 X 0.5). When the absolute granulocyte count is below 1,000, the child is considered to be neutropenic. The lower the absolute granulocyte count, the higher the risk of infection. Most treatment regimens call for an absolute granulocyte count greater than 750 or 1,000 before chemotherapy is started.

Acute Lymphocytic Leukemia (ALL)

A type of leukemia that arises from cells destined to be lymphocytes. Lymphocytes are a type of white blood cells. The defect that leads to the development of ALL is unknown. Once the cell has developed, it begins to reproduce itself. Eventually there are so many leukemic cells that there is no room for normal blood cells. Initially the cells remain in the bone marrow but eventually they spill over into the blood stream. This leads to the usual presenting symptoms of fevers, infections, bruising and bleeding, weakness, paleness, lethargy and fatigue, enlargement of the lymph nodes, spleen, and/or liver, and bone aches. ALL is treated with chemotherapy.

Acute Myelocytic Leukemia (AML)

A type of leukemia that arises from cells destined to be myelocytes. Myelocytes are a type of white blood cells. The defect that leads to the development of AML is unknown. There are seven different subtypes of myelocytes that can become malignant. The symptoms of AML are very similar to those of ALL. Some children will present with solid masses that are made up of AML cells. Other children may also have swelling of the gums. AML is treated with chemotherapy that is usually much more intensive than that used in ALL. Bone marrow transplant from a brother or sister is used for treatment if there is an available match.

Acute Promyelocytic Leukemia (APML)

A specific type of AML also known as M3. In this type of AML, the leukemic cell is more mature than in most types of AML. APML cells contain many granules that can cause problems with excess bleeding at diagnosis. A new treatment using All Trans Retinoic Acid (ATRA, a precursor of Vitamin A) has been very successful and greatly increased the cure rate for this subtype of AML.

AIDS

A disease produced by a virus, the HIV virus, which attacks the body's. The T-lymphocytes are an important part of the immune system. The attack by the virus weakens the immune system and makes the person susceptible to attack by many different viruses, bacteria, parasites and other organisms.

Anemia

A red blood cell count that is lower than expected for the child's age. Anemia can be due to many causes including bleeding, a lack of production of red cells by the bone marrow or destruction of the red cells after they are formed. The symptoms of anemia are paleness, weakness, lethargy, dizziness, decreased activity, headache, and irritability. Severe anemia from chemotherapy most often is treated with red cell transfusions.

Anticipatory Vomiting

The *knowledge* that certain treatments can *cause* vomiting can *lead* to vomiting due to the anxiety that vomiting might occur. This type of vomiting is best treated with agents that decrease anxiety.

Antiemetic

An agent that decreases the risk of vomiting.

Assent

When a minor gives official permission to proceed with a treatment.

Band

A slightly immature granulocyte. The nucleus of a band does not have *lobulations* like a mature granulocyte, but it has all of the functions of the mature cell.

Bone Marrow

The space inside the bones where all of the blood cells (red cells, white cells and platelets) are made.

Bone Marrow Aspiration

The doctor (or sometimes the nurse) sticks a special needle into a bone (usually the hipbone) and pulls out some of the bone marrow with a syringe. The material looks like thick blood but contains many bone marrow cells. The bone marrow is sent to the laboratory for special tests and examination under a microscope to see what kinds of cells are contained in the child's bone marrow.

Bone Marrow Biopsy

The doctor (or sometimes the nurse) sticks a special needle into a bone (usually the hipbone) and takes out a small piece of the bone marrow. The material is sent to the laboratory to be looked at under a microscope by a pathologist to determine an estimate of the number and kind of cells contained in the child's bone marrow.

Bone Marrow Salvage
(also called Stem Cell Salvage)

Many different cancers respond to chemotherapy, but the higher the dose, the better the chance that the cancer will be cured. The problem: doses needed to kill the cancer cells completely may also kill normal cells, especially the bone marrow cells. In a bone marrow salvage, bone marrow or another source of the cells (stem cells) that will grow to become the bone marrow cells are removed and set aside. The child then receives very high doses of chemotherapy and/or radiation. The doses of the medicines and radiation are high enough that the child's normal bone marrow would not grow back if the normal bone marrow cells were not set aside. Once the child has taken all of the chemotherapy and radiation therapy, the bone marrow (or stem cell culture) is then given back to the child in a manner similar to a blood transfusion. The cells that have been set aside find their way back to the bone marrow and begin to grow.

Bone Marrow Transplantation
(also called Stem Cell Transplantation)

This process is very similar to that used for bone marrow salvage. The difference is that the bone marrow cells of the person with cancer cannot be used because they may contain cancer cells. In a bone marrow transplantation, the marrow cells or another source of cells (stem cells) from another person are used. There are several possible sources. The best source is a matched related brother or sister. If there is no match in the family, then a match from an unrelated person might be found in the National Marrow Donor Registry, a listing of people who have volunteered to donate their bone marrow. Another possible source for bone marrow tranplantation is the blood that remains in the umbilical cord of a newborn baby. Once again, these cells need to be matched to the recipient, but the match does not have to be as close as with the other sources of bone marrow cells.

Brain Stem Glioma

The brain stem is the portion of the brain which connects the upper portions of the cerebrum with the spinal cord and peripheral nerves. A critical portion of the brain, it controls all involuntary nerve function such as breathing and heart pumping. *Glioma* cells are the cells which hold the nerve cells together. A malignant growth of the glioma cells that occurs in the brain stem is called a brain stem glioma. There are two main sections of the brain stem, the *pons* and the *medulla*. Tumors that arise in the pons are associated with dysfunction of nerves in the face and eyes as well as weakness on one side of the body. Tumors that arise in the medulla may have similar findings. The tumors are usually diagnosed with an MRI scan. If the tumor arises in the pons, it is often diagnosed and treated without a biopsy because of the delicate nature of the brain tissue of the pons. Tumors arising in the medulla can often be treated by aggressive surgery to remove the tumor. The treatment of the brain tumor gliomas that arise in the pons has usually included radiation therapy but the results have been very poor.

Brain Tumor

A tumor that arises in any part of the brain. Some types of brain tumors seen in children include *medulloblastoma, ependymoma, glioma*, and *craniopharyngioma*. Some tumors are considered benign in that they grow slowly and rarely, if ever, spread to other parts of the brain or outside of the brain. Other tumors are considered to be malignant since they grow much more rapidly and may spread to other areas. The type of tumor is often less important that the location of the tumor. A benign brain tumor growing in a critical area of the brain may be more devastating than a malignant brain tumor growing in a less important area of the brain.

Cardiopulmonary Resuscitation (CPR)

The use of special techniques to keep the air way open, to provide oxygen and to keep the heart pumping blood in a patient whose heart has stopped and who is not breathing. This technique decreases organ damage while doctors are trying to get the heart and lungs working again.

Catheter

A special plastic tube used to allow doctors to have access to a patient's blood vessels. Catheters can be placed into a small vein on a temporary basis or can be placed into large vessels on a more permanent basis depending on the needs of the patient.

Central Venous Catheter (Central Line)

A special catheter made of a soft plastic that is placed in a major blood vessel during surgery. One end is threaded through the vein into the major vein that leads into the heart. The other end is tunneled under the skin from where it exits the major blood vessel to a spot several inches away on the body. Sometimes that end of the catheter is attached to a port that is implanted under the skin. To access the port, the doctor or nurse uses a special needle called a *Hueber needle*. Blood can be drawn from the port and medicines can be given into the port. Sometimes that end of the catheter exits the skin. The catheter is closed off by a special cap. Blood can be drawn through the cap and medicines and fluids can be given back in through the catheter without the child being stuck with a needle. Both kinds of central venous catheters have advantages and disadvantages. Both increase the child's chances of infection and clotting.

Cerebellum

A portion of the brain found near the brainstem that is involved in balance. Malignant tumors that arise in this portion of the brain include *medulloblastomas* and *ependymomas*. *Cerebellar astrocytomas* are often benign tumors that can frequently be cured by surgery alone. Symptoms of cerebellar tumors include vomiting, headaches, difficulty with eye movements, and changes in balance.

Cerebrum

That portion of the brain where the major activities of the brain including thinking, memory, vision, hearing, motor movement and sensation occur. There are four major parts of the cerebrum: the frontal lobe, the parietal lobe, the temporal lobe and the occipital lobe and each is duplicated on the right and left side.

Chemotherapy

The chemical drugs used in the treatment of cancer. Most of the chemotherapy drugs work by interfering somehow in cell division. When cells are unable to divide, they die. Chemotherapy medications have a very narrow margin between their effective actions and their side effects.

Children's Cancer Group (CCG)

An international organization made up of doctors, nurses and other healthcare professionals involved in the diagnosis, treatment and follow-up of children with cancer. This organization was founded in 1955. Since its beginning, it has been responsible for caring for more than 40,000 children. More than 20,000 of those children have survived more than 5 years from the diagnosis of their cancers. The remarkable advances in the treatment of children with cancer has largely been due to the efforts of the CCG and other such organizations.

CT Scan

A special visualization technique that uses X-rays and computers to produce very accurate pictures of whatever area of the body is being imaged.

Echocardiogram

A special technique that uses sound waves to make pictures of the heart. It is an easy way for a doctor to see the flow of blood through the heart and the function of the heart valves and muscle.

Ependymoma

A type of malignant brain tumor that arises from cells that line the fluid filled portions of the brain.

Extern

A person who has not yet graduated from medical school who works in a medical environment learning how to take care of patients. An extern is always under the supervision of a medical doctor.

Faith Healer

A person who advocates the healing of human diseases through a belief in God.

GCSF

A substance produced nominally by the body that stimulates the bone marrow to make granulocytes, a type of white blood cells important in fighting bacteria. GCSF has now been made in large quantities by a few companies. It can be given subcutaneously or intravenously to people whose bone marrow is making inadequate amounts of granulocytes to shorten the time when the white blood cell count is low following chemotherapy and decrease the risk of infection.

Germ Cell Tumor

A malignant tumor that arises from cells that were supposed to become cells of the testes in boys or cells of the ovaries in girls. While many of these tumors arise in the testicle or in the ovary, they may arise in other parts of the body because germ cells sometimes get trapped in other sites during development of the embryo.

Graft Vs. Host Disease (GVHD)

This is a disease that sometimes occurs in patients who have undergone bone marrow transplantation. In the process of killing the malignant cells using very high doses of chemotherapy or radiation, the patient's immune system is severely damaged. The new cells that are given to take the place of the old bone marrow cells that have been destroyed have an intact immune system, but that immune system belongs to the donor and not to the recipient. The immune cells of the donor are activated after the new marrow begins to grow and they begin to reject the host. Graft-vs.-Host Disease. GVHD can be acute or chronic. If severe, it can result in severe skin, lung, gastrointestinal or liver problems. GHVD can also help eliminate residual malignant cells. Most patients need to take special medicines following a bone marrow transplant to decrease or eliminate the risk of GVHD.

Granulocytes
(also known as segs or neutrophils)

One of the 5 types of white blood cells. These white blood cells are usually the most common type seen. They are very important in ingesting and destroying invading bacteria. Absence or significant decrease in these white blood cells greatly increases the risk of infection.

Hepatoblastoma

This is a rare malignant tumor that arises in the liver of young children. It is associated with significant elevation of alpha-feto protein levels. Surgery in combination with chemotherapy may result in the cure of nearly 3 out of 4 children with this type of cancer.

Hodgkin's Disease

A kind of cancer of the lymph nodes. It occurs in children most commonly during the adolescent years. The most common site of involvement is the lymph nodes of the neck. Frequently the tumor will spread to the lymph nodes in the center of the chest and sometimes to the liver, spleen, and/or the lymph nodes in the abdomen. Sometimes the tumor will attack the lungs, the bone marrow or other tissues. Most young people with Hodgkin's Disease present with painless swelling that is frequently quite large and painless. The child may have unexplained weight loss, night sweats or fevers. The malignancy is treated with chemotherapy and sometimes with radiation therapy. It has a high cure rate in young people.

Home Health Care

A recent addition to the way that children with cancer are cared. Home health care companies are institutions designed to provide medical care including medications, intravenous fluids and nutrition, and hospice care that have traditionally been provided in a hospital or office setting. The large movement to use home health care that has occurred in the past 15 years is due to two reasons: the comfort and ease of receiving treatments in one's own home and the cost savings that such care produces.

Hospice

When a child's cancer is no longer responding to treatment, the parents and the child may opt to receive support, pain medication and other forms of comforting treatments during the dying process. Hospice provides this support in the patient's home or in a special center that may or may not be in a hospital. The hospice program accepts that medical treatments have done all they can to provide a cure and allows a family to deal with the reality of the disease in a dignified, peaceful environment with as little pain and as much comfort as possible. There are organized hospice programs available in most cities.

Induction

The first phase of therapy, especially therapy of leukemia. Induction is designed to bring about (induce) a remission.

Ketamine

A medicine that induces a dissociative state. The child who receives ketamine is sedated and does not respond to painful procedures or tests. The medicine has been used by burn units, emergency rooms, pediatric oncologists and other medical specialties needing to do procedures that take fairly short periods but which can be painful. Some of the children who receive this medication will have intense dreams or hallucinations. They must be watched closely while asleep and as they awaken.

Lethargy

Fatigue; a lack of energy.

Leukemia

The term comes from words that mean "white blood." The cause of the disorder is unknown, but something happens to the chromosomes of a white blood cell. If the white blood cell is destined to become a granulocyte, then the type of leukemia will be acute myelogenous leukemia. If the white blood cell is destined to become a lymphocyte, then the type of leukemia will be acute lymphocytic leukemia. Acute lymphocytic leukemia represents about 80% of all childhood leukemias. Acute myelogenous leukemia represents about 20% of all childhood leukemias. There are a few other rare types of leukemia that occur in children including chronic myelogenous leukemia and juvenile myelomonocytic leukemia.

Lumbar Puncture

See spinal tap.

Lymphocyte

Lymphocytes are one of the 5 different white blood cells. They are usually the second most common type seen in a blood count. Most lymphocytes are either B or T cells. The B cells are the lymphocytes that create antibodies. Antibodies are important in getting rid of new infections and in keeping memories of old infections so that they do not recur. T cells are important in calling other parts of the immune system into an area where an infection is occurring so that the infection can be controlled.

Lymphoma

A cancer of the lymph nodes. There are two types: Hodgkin's Disease and Non-Hodgkin's Lymphoma.

MRI (Magnetic Resonance Imaging) scan

A special type of radiological technique that uses magnets and radio waves to create pictures of the internal portions of various parts of the body. The MRI scan is a very valuable technique to identify various tumors, especially brain tumors. The machine must be housed in a special place because of the very strong magnet used to operate it. The person being scanned is placed in a narrow tube-like structure and must remain completely still during the test. The machine is very loud. Some people are very frightened by the narrow space and the noise. Younger children usually need to be sedated for the procedure.

Medulloblastoma

A brain tumor that arises from the cerebellum. The tumor occurs more commonly in children especially between the ages of 5 and 10. The most common presenting signs are headache, vomiting, balance problems and dysfunction of the nerves that go to the eyes, face and neck. The prognosis of the tumor depends on the ability of the neurosurgeon to remove the tumor and whether it has spread when it is first found.

Mucormycosis

A type of fungus that attacks people with immune problems. This fungus is now known as *Rhizopus*. This infection is very difficult to treat and very invasive and aggressive.

National Marrow Donor Program

A federally sponsored program in which people volunteer to donate their bone marrow to another person if they happen to match, even though the person is unrelated. The program was started because only about 1 of every 4 persons who needs a bone marrow transplant has a match within their family. It is possible to find a match for about 60% of people through the national marrow donor program.

Nephrologist

A doctor who specializes in the care of the kidney and kidney diseases.

Neuroblastoma

A malignant tumor that arises from cells of the sympathetic nervous system. The main site for this tumor is the adrenal gland, a very important organ that sits on top of the kidney. However, the tumor may arise in other parts of the abdomen or the back of the chest. The disease most often occurs in very young children and may even be present at birth. In children over a year of age when diagnosed, the tumor has often spread to other tissues such as the bones and the bone marrow. Neuroblastomas that are small and have not spread when found have a very good prognosis. There is a very unusual type of neuroblastoma called a type IVS that sometimes occurs in young children. Usually the primary tumor is small but there is also involvement of the liver, the bone marrow and/or the skin. Children with this type of neuroblastoma may get better without any therapy. Sometimes neuroblastomas can be associated with unusual symptoms such as unusual uncontrolled eye and body movements (known as *opsoclonus/myocionus syndrome* (or "dancing eyes/dancing feet"), or very watery diarrhea.

Most neuroblastomas present with a large mass or with pain. Neuroblastomas are treated with surgery. If the tumors are larger or if they have spread, they often need intensive chemotherapy. Some of the children with more advanced disease need to receive bone marrow or stem cell salvage procedures.

Neuropsychologist

A psychologist who specializes in the testing of brain function. Such a professional identifies specific neurological deficits or problems and helps to develop strategies to decrease or eliminate them.

Neutropenia

When the absolute granulocyte count is below 1,000, the child is considered to have neutropenia and to be neutropenic. Protection against neutropenia is best accomplished by good hand washing. Most centers have guidelines for protection of children who are neutropenic.

Neutrophil

See granulocyte.

Non-Hodgkin's Lymphomas

Malignant tumors of the lymph nodes. In children, nearly all of these tumors are considered to be disseminated (or spread throughout the body) when they are discovered. There are three types that are seen in children: lymphoblastic lymphomas; small, non-cleaved lymphomas (also known as Burkit's lymphomas); and large cell (or immunoblastic) lymphomas. Lymphoblastic lymphomas most often occur in the front part of the chest just in front of the heart. The cells resemble ALL cells. If more than 25% of the bone marrow cells are these cells, the child is considered to have ALL. The small, non-cleaved lymphomas most often arise in the tonsils or in the intestines. The large cell lymphomas can arise in the chest or in the abdomen or even in other locations.

These are highly malignant tumors but they have fairly high cure rates with modem therapies that mostly consists of chemotherapy.

Osteogenic Sarcoma

A malignant tumor that arises in the bones. This tumor occurs most commonly in teenagers. The most common site is in the bones around the knee but any bone can be involved. The most common signs of this tumor are bone pain that interferes with activity and gets worse over time and a swelling near the site of the pain. The treatment consists of chemotherapy. Surgery to remove the involved bone is essential. Most children are able to have a *limb-salvage procedure* where the involved bone is removed but special surgical techniques are used to save the limb from amputation. Special orthopedic doctors trained in these surgical techniques are necessary in order to provide the best results.

Pediatric Intensivist

A doctor who specializes in the care of children who are in a pediatric intensive care unit.

Pediatric Intensive Care Unit

An intensive care unit found in a hospital that is dedicated solely to the care of children.

Platelets

The smallest of the blood cells. Platelets are made from the bone marrow in cells known as *megakaryocytes*. The platelets circulate in the blood stream. When a hole is created in a blood vessel, the platelets get sticky. They stick to themselves and to the hole and plug up the leak. If the platelet count is low due to decreased production of the cells by the bone marrow or increased destruction of the cells after they are formed, the child will have an increased risk of bruising and bleeding. The smallest of the bruises is called *petechiae*. Larger bruises are called *purpura*. The largest braises are called *ecchymoses*.

Radiation Therapy

The use of high doses of X-rays to kill cancer cells. A special doctor, a radiation therapist, is trained to administer the radiation. When a child goes for radiation, the radiation therapist plans out the areas that are to receive the radiation. Marks are made on the child's body to map out the place where the radiation is to go every day. A small amount of radiation (a fraction) is given every day until the total amount desired has been delivered. Side effects of radiation depend on the amount and the type of normal tissue included in the radiation field.

Red Blood Cell

A type of blood cell made in the bone marrow that carries oxygen from the lungs to the tissues and carbon dioxide and other wastes from the tissues to the lungs. An inadequate number of red blood cells is called anemia.

Relapse

When the cancer or leukemia returns after a period of time when it seemed to be gone.

Remission

This term is especially used to describe the status of leukemia after a successful induction. Remission means that when the blood cells and the bone marrow are examined, it is not possible using standard microscope examinations to tell that there are any malignant cells present. Remission is not cure. In a remission, the bone marrow and blood appear to be normal but malignant cells may be present. In a cure, no malignant cells are present.

Retinoblastoma

A malignant tumor that arises in the back of the eye (or retina). Retinoblastomas occur most commonly in very young children. If they arise in both eyes or as multiple tumors in one eye, they have a genetic component. The retinoblastoma gene was one of the first cancer genes to be identified. Retinoblastomas are highly curable if discovered early. Children with retinoblastomas usually present with a white reflex or with crossed eyes. When light bounces off the back of the retina, it appears to be red. If a retinoblastoma tumor is in the way, the light that bounces off the retina appears white. That is known as the white reflex. The white reflex is most often due to a retinoblastoma although there are other conditions that can produce such a reflex.

Rhabdomyosarcoma

The most common soft tissue cancer in children. This cancer arises from the skeletal muscle. It can come from any muscle of the body so it can arise in many different locations. The outcome with the tumor is based on its histology (how it looks under the microscope), its size, whether it can be removed by a surgeon, its location, and whether it has spread to other locations when it is diagnosed. The treatment for rhabdomyosarcomas consists of surgery followed by chemotherapy. Often, radiation therapy is also used.

Segs (Segmented Cells)

See granulocyte.

Spinal Tap

The spinal cord ends near the level of the 2nd lumbar vertebrae. The spinal fluid, which flows down the center of the spinal cord from where it is made in the center of the brain, is released inside a membrane called the *dural sac*. The nerves from the end of the spinal cord travel through this fluid on their way to the lower extremity. A special needle is placed through the skin into the space between the spinal bones of the 3rd and 4th or the 4th and 5th lumbar vertebrae. Fluid is collected and sent to the lab for special tests.

White Blood Cell

A type of cell made in the bone marrow that is extremely important in helping the body fight infections. There are 5 types of white blood cells: the *granulocytes*, the *lymphocytes*, the *monocytes*, the *eosinophils*, and the *basophils*. See granulocyte and lymphocyte for more information on these types of cells. The monocytes are important for cleaning up some of the debris created by the fight against various infections. In addition, monocytes help wall off certain organisms so they cannot invade other parts of the body. It takes monocytes 2-3 days to develop in the bone marrow before they are released into the blood stream. It takes granulocytes 7-10 days to do so. Monocytes appear first during recovery so the presence of monocytes can be a sign that a child with neutropenia is beginning to recover. The eosinophils are important in all allergy and parasitic infections. The basophils may be important in the inflammatory process.

Wilm's Tumor

A malignant kidney tumor that tends to occur in young children. Much like retinoblastoma, those with Wilm's Tumors in both kidneys carry a genetic abnormality. Most often children with Wilm's Tumor present with large masses in their abdomens, abdominal pain, or blood in the urine. High blood pressure or elevations in the red blood cell count can also be due to Wilm's Tumor. The prognosis of Wilm's Tumor is related to the size of the tumor, the tumor histology (how it looks to the pathologist under the microscope) and whether it has spread when it is found. The treatment of the tumor consists of surgery and chemotherapy. Radiation therapy is sometimes used as well.

Bibliography

Bain, Lisa J. *A Parent's Guide to Childhood Cancer*. Dell. New York, NY. 1998.

Baker, Lynn. S. *You and Leukemia: A Day at a Time*. W. B. Saunders Co. Philadelphia, PA. 1988.

Bracken, Jeanne Munn. *Children With Cancer: A Comprehensive Guide for Parents*. Oxford University Press. New York, NY. 1986.

Fleonar, John. *Shannon: A Book for Parents of Children With Leukemia*. Hawthor Books. Binghamptom, NY. 1975.

Fromer, Margot Joan. *Surviving Childhood Cancer*. New Harbinger Publications. Oakland, CA. 1998.

Hobbs, N. and Perrin J.B. *Issues in the Care of Children with Chronic Illness*. Jossey-Bass Publishers. San Francisco, CA. 1988.

Keene, N. *Childhood Leukemia: A Guide for Families, Friends and Caregivers*, O'Reilly and Associates, 1997.

Krementz, J. *How It Feels To Fight For Your Life*. Little, Brown and Company, 1989.

Kushner, Harold S. *When Bad Things Happen to Good People*. Schocken Books. New York, NY. 1989.

Kubler-Ross, Elizabeth, *On Children and Death*. New York, NY. MacMillan.1983.

Kushner, Harold. *When Bad Things Happen to Good People*,

Lazlo, John, M.D. *The Cure of Childhood Leukemia: Into The Age of Miracles*, Rutgers University Press. New Brunswick, NJ. 1995.

Pringle, Terry. *This Is the Child*. Random House. New York, NY. 1983.

Saunds, Lynn S. *You and Leukemia: A Day at a Time*. Orlando, FL. 1988.

Schwartz, C.L.; Hobbie, W.L.; Constantine L.S.; Ruccione, K.S. *Survivors of Childhood Cancer: Assessment and Management*, Mosby-Year Book Inc. 1994.

Truman, J.T. van Eys, J. Pochedly C. (eds.): *Human Values in Pediatric Hematology/Oncology*. Praeger. 1986.

Tucker, Jonathan B. *Ellie: A Child's Fight Against Leukemia*. Holt, Rinehart and Winston, New York, NY. 1982.

Index

If You Liked This Book

If you liked this book, please tell your friends about it, or better yet, get a copy for them and your library. While most of our books are available through bookstores, not all booksellers carry our titles. Call us at (800) 324-5663, e-mail, fax or write, or find this book on the web at http://www.emeraldink.com and its various links. Our goal: books good enough to read! Other titles available from Emerald Ink:

Business & Home

Debt Control, Chris Richards, 1-885373- 19-8.
Start A Business Without Borrowing,
D. Kelly Irvin, 1-885373-06-6 (now only through publisher).
Understanding & Reducing Your Home Electric Bill,
Richard L. Hepburn, MS, 1-885373-01-5.

Fiction:

My Father's Son, Alex Keaton, 1-885373-24-4.

History/Travel

China Mailbag Unsealed, Lou Glist, 1-885373-21-X.
Reflections of A Rotarian, Jack Pearce, 1-885373-04-X.

Health

A Time for Alzheimer's, Florence Baurys, R.N. 1885373-13-9.
Conquering Kid's Cancer, Ken Lazaraus, MD, 1-885373-22-8.
How I Conquered Cancer, Eric Gardiner, 1-885373-11-2.
(Audio 1-555373-16-3).

Spiritual

Holy Man, Holy War, Fred Berry, 1-885373-10-4.
The Lazarus Adventure: Stepping Into the Light,
Judi Williams, 1-885373-25-2.
Mary of Galilee, Woodard, 1-885373-23-6.
To Hell And Back, Don Brubaker, Audio 1-885373-17-1
When Ego Dies—A Compilation of Near-Death and Mystical Conversion
Stories, 1-885373-07-4.

Emerald Ink Publishing
9700 Almeda-Genoa Road #502
Houston, Texas 77075
(800) 324-5663, Fax 713 946-6066
E-mail emerald@emeraldink.com • http://www.emeraldink.com